Ayurveda

Unleashing the Power of the Ayurvedic Diet, Yoga, Meditation, and Aromatherapy for Healing and Balancing Your Chakras

Your Free Gift (only available for a limited time)

Thanks for getting this book! If you want to learn more about various spirituality topics, then join Mari Silva's community and get a free guided meditation MP3 for awakening your third eye. This guided meditation mp3 is designed to open and strengthen ones third eye so you can experience a higher state of consciousness. Simply visit the link below the image to get started.

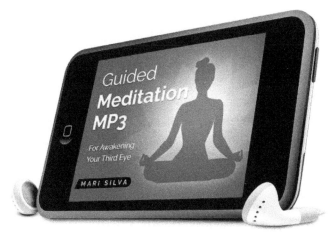

https://spiritualityspot.com/meditation

Contents

Introduction

Ayurveda is one of the oldest healthcare systems in the world. This ancient philosophy has its roots in ancient India, dating to over 5000 years. It essentially offers a primary framework for caring for the physical body to improve your overall health and internal balance. A primary belief in Ayurveda is that all individuals are unique and, your path to health is unique too. Even though it is not a new science, its ancient wisdom is ideal in every aspect of your life today. When you concentrate on healing the connection between the mind and body and by becoming conscious of your lifestyle choices, you can improve your overall health.

Several things in life are beyond your control, but your health and wellbeing are not among these things. Ayurveda is a holistic system that offers all the guidance you need to change your lifestyle and diet to improve your overall health. By bringing together your body, mind, soul, and senses, you create an internal harmony that is the key to improve your sense of wellbeing and health.

This book will teach you about the history and origin of Ayurveda, its principles, and the different benefits it offers. You will discover the five elements and three doshas in Ayurveda and their importance. This book introduces you to the eight Ayurveda branches, practical tips to follow the Ayurvedic diet, and the relationship between the seven chakras and Ayurveda. Besides this, you will learn about the importance of yoga and meditation in Ayurvedic philosophy and practical tips to include these practices in your life.

By following the Ayurvedic detox, you can detoxify your body internally and improve your overall health. This book will act as your guide and offer all the information you need to successfully merge the ancient practice of Ayurveda into your daily life to optimize the benefits it offers. Once you are armed with all this information, you can heal and balance your body internally. Ayurveda holds the key to improving the quality of your life and your overall health.

Are you curious to learn more about all this? Are you excited to step into the world of Ayurveda? If yes, let's get started immediately.

Chapter 1: What is Ayurveda?

The Sanskrit word Ayurveda combines two words - Ayur and Veda. Ayur means life, while Veda means knowledge or science. When you put these words together, Ayurveda translates to the science or knowledge of life. It is founded on the idea that the body, mind, and spirit are intricately connected with everything that happens within and around us. This holistic approach to health is based on the concept of universal connectedness.

Ayurveda is believed to be the mother of all healing, and its knowledge originated in India over 5000 years ago. It includes several natural methods and remedies to promote wellness of the body, mind, and soul. The primary principle on which Ayurveda rests is the interconnectedness of the body and mind. It suggests that the mind has the power to transform and heal an individual's entire being.

An important aspect of Ayurveda that differentiates it from other health practices is it considers that no two individuals are alike, so the treatment needs to be different too. According to Ayurvedic practices, the treatment ideal for every person depends on the state of their doshas. You will learn about all this in the later chapters.

History and Origin

According to the sacred texts known as Vedas, it's believed that the Rishis or seers in India received all knowledge about Ayurveda from the Hindu gods over 5000 years ago. The information to attain a well-balanced and healthy life was recorded in these Vedas. Vedas are among the oldest forms of known literature. They were written in Sanskrit and are considered sacred Hindu texts. Vedas include the records of different revelations, knowledge, and the ancient wisdom sages obtained through different sources.

There are four Vedas, namely the Rig Veda, Yajur Veda, Sama Veda, and the Atharva Veda. The Atharva Veda was believed to have been compiled around 900 BCE. It includes information about ancient medicinal practices, described comprehensively and systematically. The available knowledge of Ayurveda comes from the Atharva Veda.

Now, let's go back to mythology once again to understand the origin of Ayurveda. According to Hindu mythology, three Gods are responsible for the creation and maintenance of the universe. They are known as the Trimurti. Of these, the Lord Brahma plays the role of the creator, and he is believed to have created Ayurveda. His knowledge about Ayurveda was passed on to his son, Daksha Prajapati, who passed it on to Ashwini Kumaras, the twin Vedic gods. The information Ashwini Kumaras obtained was presented to the god Indra. Lord Indra had three physicians in his court, Acharya Bharadwaj, Acharya Divodas Dhanvantari, and Acharya Kashyapa. These three physicians were presented with the knowledge of Ayurveda. Agnivesha, a disciple of Bharadwaj, developed the primary Ayurvedic text about internal medicine based on his teacher's teachings. Acharya Charak, a disciple of Agnivesha, revisited and revised his body of work and passed it on to his disciples. This is how the knowledge of Ayurveda is believed to have been introduced to mankind.

Basic Principles of Ayurveda

Before you learn more about healing your body, mind, and soul using Ayurveda, you need to learn its basic principles. By remembering these simple principles, all the information in the subsequent chapters will make more sense.

According to Ayurvedic teachings, the fundamental energies in the universe regulate all the natural processes that take place within it. Three fundamental universal energies influence events at a microcosmic and macrocosmic level. The different energies responsible for all the interactions between planets, stars, and galaxies operate within the human body too. These three energies are known as Tridosa or Tridosha in Sanskrit.

All the information and wisdom about Ayurveda flows from an absolute source known as the Paramatma or the absolute being. Our health is the amalgamation of energy, which acts through the laws of nature or Prakriti. Ayurveda helps balance individuals and nature. It ensures that we live our lives based on nature's laws to optimize our overall health and wellbeing.

Instead of concentrating on creating treatments that focus only on individual symptoms, Ayurveda offers a holistic approach to health and healing. Its primary focus is to create and maintain a balance between all the life energies to promote your health and healing.

Since we all have specific constitutional differences, various regimes are required for varying people. Even if two individuals have similar external symptoms, their internal energies' constitution and composition can vary. This is why Ayurveda offers personalized and customized remedies, depending on the individual's energy composition.

The holistic approach of Ayurveda concentrates on maintaining the connection between the body and mind. It offers several tools and information that prompts us to concentrate on the subtler aspects of our body, mind, and spirit. When there is a fragmentation of these things or discord and imbalance, it manifests itself as poor mental, physical, or emotional health. By paying attention to the complex yet crucial mind-body connection, Ayurveda helps restore a sense of harmony and wholeness.

Several treatments, exercises, and therapies suggested by Ayurveda help rebalance all the five elements and three doshas of the body and its senses. For instance, meditation, exercise, and repetition of mantras are used to balance the mind's elements. You will learn about all this in the following chapters.

There are five essential elements in Ayurveda, and they are known as panchabhutas. They are space, water, air, fire, and earth. These five elements manifest themselves within our bodies along with three primary forces known as doshas or tridoshas, which are Vata, pitta, and Kapha. Combining these three doshas helps create, maintain, assimilate, and destroy various cells and tissues within our bodies. The unique combination of these three doshas a person is born with is known as Prakriti or the fundamental constitution. Since we all have different Prakriti, the combination of diet, exercise, and cleansing or rebuilding therapies required to optimize our overall health differs.

Applications of Ayurveda

Even though the concept of Ayurveda is not new, its applications are still as relevant to modern life as they were when it was introduced. If you wonder whether Ayurveda is for you or want to learn about the different benefits it offers, read on.

Reduce Stress

The Vedic knowledge from which Ayurveda was obtained stresses the interconnection between Ayurvedic knowledge and yoga. Both these concepts and philosophies show the intricate relationship between the universe and our consciousness. Several Ayurvedic techniques and methods are specifically designed to reduce stress. Since the modern world we live in has become synonymous with stress, learning to handle it is essential for your overall health and wellbeing. For instance, Ayurveda talks about the importance of meditation and dinacharya. The concept of dinacharya is simple. It refers to a daily routine based on cycles of nature. It refers to the practice of waking up at sunrise. Remember the age-old adage by Benjamin Franklin, "Early to bed, early to rise makes a man healthy, wealthy and wise?" It turns out, this saying is true. Establishing a sleep-wake cycle in sync with the sunrise and sunset helps readjust the circadian rhythm. Once your circadian rhythm is in sync with daylight and nighttime, your ability to sleep and wake up on time becomes more effortless. Besides this, Ayurveda also talks about the importance of meditation. Meditation helps reduce stress and combat the production of stress hormones. It is also believed that meditation teaches mindfulness watch is vital for making the most of every minute available. You will learn about all these things in the next chapters.

Weight Loss

An essential benefit of Ayurveda is it helps in natural weight loss that doesn't harm your physical or emotional health. By following an Ayurvedic diet, you can lose weight and fat and maintain these results. Since it is sustainable in the long run, let go of any worries about it being a crash diet. By following an Ayurvedic diet, you can detoxify your body from within, promoting the removal of any excess fat present within the tissues while purifying your body of all the toxins building up. It can reduce the levels of cholesterol while promoting blood circulation. You will learn more about the Ayurvedic diet later in this book.

Promote Self-Understanding

Ayurveda is based on the concept that every individual is unique. All the suggestions it offers can be personalized and tailor-made according to your approach to life. It encourages self-love instead of engaging in unhealthy and undesirable comparisons. By identifying and recognizing your personal needs, it becomes easier to heal yourself. The simple principle of everyone being unique is based on the concept of body types and personality characteristics identified as doshas. The three doshas in Ayurveda - Vata, pitta, and Kapha - are present in everyone in varying proportions. By recognizing all this, you get a better understanding of yourself as an individual.

A Holistic Approach to Health

In Ayurveda, it's believed that you and your environment need to be in complete harmony for optimum health. When there is an imbalance, it harms your health. Whether it is anxiety or any other health problem, it is all due to an imbalance within the body. These imbalances do not occur overnight, and Ayurveda teaches you to prevent them or slow down their processes.

See the Bigger Picture

According to Ayurveda, nature is made of five elements or Panchabhutas: space, air, water, fire, and earth. These elements are constantly interacting with each other and are responsible for life. For instance, fire can manifest itself as various health problems ranging from inflammation to indigestion or even present itself as a difficult emotion such as anger or rage. Earth is associated with stubbornness, loyalty, and the health of the bones. Similarly, the other elements also present themselves in your life, externally and internally. By recognizing these elements and the meaning they represent, you can work toward reestablishing a life based on the concept of harmony.

Clear Your Energy

We live in a world where we are constantly overwhelmed by different tasks. Whether it is our internal or external environment, our senses are constantly thrown into overdrive. By recalibrating your mental and physical surroundings, you can clear your energy. By improving your self-understanding, Ayurveda gives you a chance to understand what is and is not working for you. This understanding helps create space for more desirable things while eliminating unnecessary clutter. Whether it is the Ayurvedic diet to cleanse your body from within or the practice of meditation to get rid of mental clutter, Ayurveda helps cleanse your energy.

Better Cellular Health

Ayurveda is believed to promote your health at a cellular level. It recalibrates your body settings and increases its ability to heal itself from within. Your body has an internal mechanism known as autophagy that helps maintain cellular health and balance. Autophagy helps eliminate and repair any undesirable toxins while improving the health of cells within the body. When this process works properly, your health is optimal. The simplest way to do this is by paying attention to three aspects of your life: diet, exercise, and sleep. Ayurveda offers guidance about all these things to improve your overall sense of wellbeing.

Reduce the Buildup of Toxins

Most of us are guilty of consuming unhealthy diets rich in processed foods, additives, and many ingredients devoid of nutrition. When you repeatedly consume such food, you are depriving your body of vital nutrients required for health and filling it up with undesirable toxins. A common toxin known as ama builds up in your digestive system. Ama translates to a waste product. When you regularly load up on foods damaging to your body, the buildup of these toxins will increase, causing a significant imbalance between your body, mind, and spirit. By following the simple practices of Ayurveda and the Ayurvedic diet, you concentrate on clean eating. This reduces the buildup of these toxins. When these toxins are removed from the body, your internal system starts functioning like it is supposed to.

Importance of Sanskrit

The traditional script of Ayurveda is written in Sanskrit. Sanskrit is considered the language of the gods. The poetic verses of Ayurveda were initially passed down through generations based only on memorization of sacred scriptures. It was only when this knowledge traveled beyond India's borders that it was translated into other languages. The traditional Indian character of Ayurveda is still intact, which is why Sanskrit plays an important part in it. There are several Ayurvedic terms you need to get acquainted with, such as doshas, Prakriti, panchabhutas, and so on. Even if you do not get the pronunciation right, understanding these Sanskrit words increases your understanding of Ayurveda and its application.

You can't learn the concepts of Ayurveda without using Sanskrit. The term panchakarma in Sanskrit refers to a cleansing process. Literal translation aside, English terms hardly do any justice to the complexities of the treatments. Also, certain Sanskrit words don't translate well into English, and their true meaning is lost in translation. Another important reason why sticking to Sanskrit while learning Ayurveda is important is that some Sanskrit concepts do not exist in western culture.

Understanding the root words of terms used in Ayurveda makes it easier to enhance your understanding of this holistic philosophy. For instance, hrdroga is a Sanskrit word used to describe heart diseases. It is made of two words: hrd, which means heart, and roga, which means disease. You don't have to worry about learning a new language. All the information in this book has been translated for your convenience. Spending a little time learning the Sanskrit pronunciations and words will magnify the benefits of Ayurveda.

Chapter 2: The Significance of Doshas and the Five Elements

Some say that the universe and everything within it is made of the five great elements or the Panchamahabhuta. Pancha means five, maha means great, and bhuta refers to elements. Everything present in the cosmos, including living beings, is influenced by these elements. These five elements manifest themselves as three primary energy sources within the body known as tridoshas. Let's learn more about these concepts and their importance.

Understand the Five Elements

Ayurvedic teachings, principles, and philosophies are based on the idea that the cosmos is made of the Pancha maha bhutas or the five significant elements. These elements are ether or Akash, air or Vayu, fire or Agni, water or Jal, and earth or Prithvi. Each element represents an idea fundamental to the existence of matter and nature itself. They are essentially the building blocks of matter and energy that exist in nature. Unless you understand these five elements, you can't understand how Ayurveda works or the human body's composition.

The Pancha maha bhuta is believed to have originated from the Pancha tanmatra. The Sanskrit word tanmatra refers to the subtle essence of our senses. There are five senses known to us. Every element is an amalgamation of different tanmatra, but they usually show predominance for one. The five senses or Pancha tanmatra are sound or shabda, touch or sparsha, taste or rasa, vision or roopa, and smell or gandha. As you can see, each of these tanmatras is associated with a specific sensory organ.

Each element is associated with a component and a specific function. For instance, the elements are associated with tissues and their function within the physical body. They are related to your personality and basic traits mentally and spiritually, holding the key to unlocking the secrets of creation itself and the immense wisdom of the cosmos.

Let's learn about each of these elements and the role they play in our lives.

Ether

Of all the maha Pancha bhutas, ether or Akash is considered the subtlest. The Tanmatra of ether originates from shabda or sound. It refers to the primordial space, which results in vibrations that create sounds within the ears, so ether and sound are inseparable elements. The sensory organ associated with ether is the ear. Another organ associated with ether is the mouth because it is the organ of action. If there are any imbalances in how ether functions within the body, it results in hearing trouble and communication issues, especially the loss of your voice. This element is also present between all the cells and in a space present within the body. Space between the lungs, bladder, intestines, or even the blood vessels is filled with ether. The common characteristic traits associated with this personality include imagination, subtlety in thinking, and dreamlike quality. These individuals can be elusive and passive.

Air

The element of air or Vayu is believed to have evolved from ether itself. Air is created whenever the potential within any space or ether becomes active. It is a representation of motion and every other force or movement that results from it. The tanmatra associated with air or Vayu is known as sparsha. Sparsha is the sense of touch. The experience of touch is considered subtle. There exists an inseparable relationship between touch and air. We experience touch via our skin. So, the sensory organ associated with air is skin. Hands are the organs of action because we reach out and touch things using them.

The air we breathe is associated with the air present in our body. This is recognized as the primary source of life, according to ancient rishis. It is synonymous with life energy or prana. Depending on the direction of movement, the air is usually described in five forms. These five forms are inward or prana, outward or vyana, upward or udhana, downward or apana, and the centralizing or stabilizing force known as Samana. All these things are known as pranas and vayus. Air is present within the body in the form of motion, helping with respiration, communication of nerve impulses, circulation of blood, body movements, and thought flow. Any issue associated with tactile perception or the inability to hold on to your thoughts is due to the imbalance caused by this element. Those with a strong air element are agile and move and think quickly. They are enthusiastic and cheerful.

Fire

The space that fire needs to burn is provided by ether, while air gives it the capacity to continue burning. Fire or Agni is the third element created from ether and air. The Sun offers the energy earth requires, while fire offers the energy our body needs to keep going. The tanmatra of vision or roopa is the origination for fire. Roopa is associated with color and form. These result from our perception. Fire is considered the primordial form of light, vision, and our sense of perception. It gives us the light required to perceive things. Our eyes help us receive and perceive everything that takes place around us. The sensory organs associated with Agni are our eyes.

If there are any disturbances within this element, it results in disorders of visual perception. We use our feet to act on everything we see. Our feet help change our direction, the intensity of our progress, and what we do. All these things are based on our perception. If the eyes are the sensory organs associated with this element, the organ of action for fire is related to our feet. Fire represents the power to transform oneself; it stands for heat, light, metabolism, and the energy one experiences. Those with a dominant fire element are adventurous, confident, brave, motivated, progressive in their thinking, and display leadership traits. They are young at heart and are always eager to go after their goals and dreams.

Water

The fourth element is jal, apas, or water. This element comes into existence due to the fire present within us. When the air becomes dense because of fire, it results in creating water. Water protects our body and gives the basic nourishment it requires to function optimally. It protects us from the heat of the fire, dilution of ether, and the unevenness of air. If the fire causes pain and inflammation, water soothes it.

The first element we can taste is water. The tanmatra of water is rasa or taste. It is not representative of the taste itself but the experience it provides. Depending on how water manifests itself, the taste also differs. Any disorder associated with the inability to taste is due to an imbalance in this element. The tanmatra of rasa is manifested through the tongue. The sensory organ associated with this element is the tongue. Taste buds work only when there's saliva or water present. The absence of this element takes away our ability to taste. Our body also expels water through the urethra. The urethra is the organ of action associated with jal or apas. Compassion and empathy are the dominating emotions associated with this element, and water is the elemental representation of our feelings.

Earth

The fifth element is known as earth or Prithvi. Prithvi contains the essence of all the other four elements. Earth's space to exist comes from the ether, its subtle movements are promoted by air, fire is an element present within it, and water acts as a bridge between the solid and gaseous matters. This element represents the universe and lends form to our being. It is the element of creation and acts as a conduit for all the other elements to flow through.

The tanmatra of Prithvi is gandha or smell. If gandha helps us experience a smell, then earth gives up the ability to experience it within our body. The organ through which smell manifests itself is the nose. The nose is the sensory organ associated with Prithvi. The balance of this element is regulated through the process of consumption and defecation. The organ of action associated with Prithvi is the rectum. Those with potent earth element love stability are reliable and methodical, but they can also be stubborn to a certain degree.

Each element evolves into the next. If all elements originate from Akash, they are contained within Prithvi.

All About the Doshas

Ayurveda is based on healing a person according to their emotional, physical, and spiritual constitution. As mentioned earlier, Ayurvedic philosophy suggests the world is made of five elements. All these five elements constantly send energy. The energy patterns present themselves in every cell, tissue, and organ within the body, known as doshas. Doshas handle all our body processes, functions, feelings, and thoughts. There are three doshas present, and we are all a unique combination of them. Even though they're all present in us, their composition varies from one individual to another. This constitution of doshas is determined at our time of conception. As you go through different life phases, these doshas fluctuate according to your diet, environment, and several other factors. When they are not in balance, they harm our physical, mental, and emotional health.

The three doshas are Vata, Pitta, and Kapha. Vata is associated with the wind during Pitta with fire and Kapha with water. The unique combination of all these doshas makes us different from one another. We all have a primary or dominant dosha that essentially makes our constitution. Let's learn more about these three doshas, their function, and how to balance them.

Vata Dosha

This dosha is associated with the quality of space and air. It is the primary force of communication within the body. Just like the wind blows, it affects everything else, including the other two doshas.

This dosha governs all forms of movement. Whether it is the movement of the body, expression, circulation of blood, or even elimination of waste, Vata regulates at all. It also governs the functioning of our nervous system and immune system. Those with a dominant Vata dosha usually are slender with low body weight. They are thin and usually have dry skin, cold hands, and feet, and are susceptible to poor blood circulation. Individuals with a dominant Vata dosha are dynamic, quickly adapt to change, and like change.

When this dosha is well balanced, it brings a sense of comfort associated with all movement. A balanced Vata dosha implies regular breathing, a good appetite, and regular bowel movements. It handles your sense of positivity, enthusiasm, innovation, and a calm mind. When there is an excess of Vata in the body, it results in numbness of extremities, indigestion, insomnia, dehydration, dry skin, pain, and a tendency to lose weight. On the other hand, you tend to become scared, anxious, and lazy if there isn't sufficient Vata in your body. It increases the risk of arthritis, osteoporosis, and other disorders associated with movement.

The simplest way to balance Vata energy is by bringing a sense of stability and warmth into your life. Warmth over here refers to it in the literal sense. By staying warm, maintaining a regular sleeping schedule, and following a Vata dosha diet, you can rebalance this energy.

A Vata dosha diet is rich in foods with a moderately heavy texture warm. Increase your consumption of warm soups, milk, stews, hot cereals, freshly baked bread, water, nuts, cream, and butter. Herbal teas can also add the warmth your body needs to rebalance its Vata energy. Warm beverages, including warm water, will help. Sweet fruits are believed to be ideal for a Vata diet. Besides this, avoid all cold foods while working on balancing this dosha. Cold foods, including iced beverages, salads, and raw vegetables, need to be avoided as much as possible.

Pitta Dosha

The Pitta dosha helps stabilize Vata and Kapha doshas. These two doshas handle hormone regulation, digestive processes, and body metabolism. This energy's primary purpose is to regulate your heartbeat, body temperature, skin health, hormonal levels, sense of perception, and thirst, and your digestion, and liver function. Individuals with dominant Pitta dosha usually have medium weight and height and delicate skin. They are charismatic, charming, and have a keen eye for attention to detail. Pitta-dominant individuals are good communicators, sharp-witted, and efficient decision-makers.

When this energy is well balanced in your body, it helps maintain a healthy appetite, stabilizes hormone production, improves your complexion and skin health, maintains your eyesight, lends courage, and regulates your intelligence. On the downside, when there is an excess of Pitta energy in your body, it makes you overeat, causes heartburn, triggers fever and skin rashes, increases blood pressure, and leaves a bitter taste in the mouth. When there is less Pitta energy, it increases Vata and Kapha doshas. A combination of these two things reduces your body temperature while resulting in poor digestion. It can also manifest itself as irritation, frustration, and anger.

By following a Pitta dosha diet, consuming healthy and wholesome meals, and choosing cooler foods, you can balance this energy. A Pitta dosha diet is rich in cold and refreshing foods during hot weather seasons, such as ice cream, milk, and cold salads. Those with unbalanced Pitta dosha should choose plant-based foods, grains, dairy products, and herbal teas. Besides this, avoid oily and spicy foods such as sour cream, chili peppers, pickles, and cheese. Even acidic foods such as alcohol, nuts, hot spices, hot beverages, and honey need to be avoided while on this diet. Any foods or beverages that cool down your body will benefit the Pitta dosha.

Kapha Dosha

The Kapha energy holds all the cells together, forming muscles, bones, and fat. It is believed to improve the function of your brain, lungs, joints, and heart. It is also responsible for the stomach's protective lining. Usually, those with a dominant Kapha dosha have broad hips and shoulders, thick hair, and oily skin. Besides that, they have great stamina, a stable appetite, and good digestion. When this dosha's energy is well balanced, it improves your physical and mental strength and stamina. If there is too much of this dosha, it results in poor digestion, an increased desire to sleep, congestion, and a wet cough. It can cause an increased risk of diabetes, obesity, cardiovascular disorders, and high cholesterol levels if left unregulated.

By increasing your physical activity, staying warm and avoiding much dampness, and following a Kapha dosha diet, you can rebalance this dosha. The Kapha dosha diet includes foods that are dry, light, and warm. Increase your intake of spicy and warm foods, especially during the cold weather. Avoid foods too fatty or sweet.

You will learn more about the Ayurvedic diet in the later chapters.

Importance of Doshas

Are you wondering why it is important to learn about doshas? Ayurveda is based on the belief that all individuals are unique. This stems from our unique internal composition of doshas. By understanding the doshas, you can customize a diet and make helpful lifestyle choices to enhance your overall sense of wellbeing. Here are the different benefits of understanding your doshas, according to Ayurveda.

Customize Your Diet

Did you ever wonder why a certain diet seems to work for others when it doesn't work for you? If this has happened, it's probably because of your dosha constitution. Understanding your dosha makes it easier to select foods that strengthen and stabilize your internal elemental constitution. Instead of worrying about all the calories you consume, it's better to concentrate on consuming foods that harmonize all the different elements present within. By doing this, you can avoid making any unhealthy food choices while working with your body's metabolism. This is one reason why the diet works for some, it doesn't work for others.

Understand Your Emotional Responses

Your dominant dosha guides your emotional responses. Never underestimate the relationship between the emotional and elemental composition of the human body. Whether you are hotheaded, a pushover, or aloof, these are not just colloquial expressions. The different doshas that accumulate within your body manifest themselves emotionally – for instance, your irritability and anger increase when there is too much Agni present in the body.

Similarly, anxiety and worry increase if too much Vayu and Akash exist within. When there is an accumulation of water and earth elements, you feel unmotivated, stuck in a rut, and even depressed. Each of these three doshas is associated with different elements. By understanding all this, you get a better insight into the elemental composition of your emotions. This knowledge will better show you what is causing your emotional responses. Once you know the cause, you have better chances of regulating them. How can you possibly fix something when you are not aware of its source?

Better Insight into Money Matters

It might sound a little incredulous to believe, but money is also a type of energy. The different elements present in your physiological constitution determine how you spend this energy. For instance, Vata is governed by the elements of air and space. These two elements venture into the financial domain, too. Individuals with a dominant Vata dosha usually are not focused on long-term financial goals, spend their money quickly, and save little.

On the other hand, those with a dominant pitta dosha are extremely good planners and like planned luxuries and self-development. This brings us to Kapha, who is the exact opposite of Vata dosha with financial matters. Kapha holds on to the money dearly and always saves for a rainy day. Even though they're good at saving, they can go a little overboard and are often described as misers. By understanding your dosha, you get a better insight into your saving and spending habits. These two things come in handy while creating financial plans.

Spend Your Time Wisely

Did you ever practice a self-care routine that left you more exhausted than you were earlier? Perhaps you attended an event that left you more drained? If yes, it's probably because the event you chose was not the one your predominant dosha needed. Your preference for self-care and how you spend free time is associated with your dosha. By understanding any existing imbalance within your dosha, you can choose restorative activities that help rebalance your mental, physical, and emotional states.

An individual with Vata energy will love to spend time outdoors and have chats by the bonfire, while Pitta prefers social gatherings and trips to the seaside. Any activity based on movement and offers motivation appeals to the Kapha energy. Once you understand the dosha, it becomes easier to find an activity that helps enhance your overall sense of wellbeing while restoring your energy field.

A Holistic Approach to Beauty

Depending on your dosha or any imbalance of dosha in the body, the skincare regime can be customized. Understanding your dosha's different properties and how it's expressed through your skin, using the right supplements and elements to enhance your skin health becomes easier. By doing this, your skin becomes more resistant at performing its job as a barrier that protects your body from toxins and pollutants. Besides this, you can also enhance its radiance.

For instance, individuals with more Vata energy often have dry skin, while Pitta has a higher risk of redness and inflammation. Individuals with Vata will benefit from greater hydration, while Pitta individuals will need something that helps calm and soothe their skin. By familiarizing yourself with specific doshas in the body, developing a conscious beauty and skincare regime becomes easier.

Personalized Exercise Program

The exercise routine also varies depending on the doshas. Customizing your workouts and finding one that works well with your body's metabolism becomes easier by understanding your doshas. Individuals with a Vata body type usually have thin and light frames, while Pittas have a strong physique. The ideal exercise for the Vata body types is anything that increases their strength, while Pitta needs higher physical intensity exercises. An ideal exercise for Pitta doshas is swimming, which helps reduce the internal flames in their body. The Kapha types usually have a tough time starting an exercise regime. The perfect exercise for them concentrates on improving their cardiovascular fitness.

Accepting Your Body

By now, you must realize that we are all a unique combination of all five elements. Depending on the extent to which these elements are present, your physical characteristics vary. Instead of a singular approach to beauty, Ayurveda offers various customization options depending on an individual's elemental composition. Vata individuals have a thin and delicate body frame while pitta leans toward strong and sleek frames and Kapha all about curves and fullness. By understanding your dosha, you are acknowledging all the unique characteristics and traits it comes with. We live in a world that is obsessed with the idea of perfection and idealizes specific body types. Instead, Ayurveda acknowledges and embraces all your unique properties and increases your self-acceptance. Without self-acceptance, practicing self-love is impossible. Understanding your dosha or elemental composition enables self-acceptance. Understanding your natural expression makes it easier to follow a diet or exercise regime that fits your unique needs.

Understanding your dosha offers a holistic approach to health that considers your uniqueness. By understanding the elemental expression of your body, mind, and spirit, you can take conscious actions to create a life that is stable, well balanced, and focused on health. Ayurveda helps you choose a holistic approach to wellbeing.

Chapter 3: The Eight Branches of Ayurveda

Ayurveda is so much more than just understanding the different doshas and elemental composition of the body. Ashtanga Ayurveda is the term used to refer to the eight branches or limbs of Ayurveda. Ashta means eight in Sanskrit, and Anga means limbs or branches. Ashtanga Ayurveda refers to the different specializations present in Ayurveda. The knowledge of branches of science is what ashtanga Ayurveda is all about. It's about studying a specific branch of science and then graduating to a different level within the same science under different teachers. During the olden days, those studying Ayurveda moved from one campus to another to specialize in a branch in which they were interested. This system is similar to the undergrad, post-grad, and Ph.D. system we have in modern education.

The eight Ayurveda branches are Kaya chikitsa, Bala chikitsa, Graha chikitsa, Urdhwanga chikitsa, Shalya Tantra, Damshtra chikitsa, Jara chikitsa, and Visha chikitsa. Do not be overwhelmed by all these Sanskrit names. Once you understand each of these, your knowledge of Ayurveda will automatically increase. It also helps you see the similarities between modern medicine and ancient holistic knowledge of Ayurveda.

Kaya Chikitsa

The first branch of Ashtanga Ayurveda is known as Kaya chikitsa. Kaya chikitsa is the Sanskrit term for general medicine. Kaya means body, and chikitsa means treatment. It is associated with diagnosing and treating widespread diseases, including diabetes, skin disorders, and rheumatoid arthritis. The most crucial scripture available on Kaya chikitsa is Charaka Samhita. It discusses the primary principles of treatment and different therapies and detoxification methods used to improve your health. This is a natural and holistic treatment based on the belief that an individual's physical body results from several psychosomatic interactions that continuously take place, and any disorders or illnesses caused are due to imbalance in the three doshas. If there is an imbalance due to Vata, Pitta, or Kapha doshas, it could be caused by the mind or the body's tissues. Toxin deposits are known as ama.

This holistic approach toward health identifies the root cause of an illness. All Ayurvedic therapies are based on the concept of Agni. Agni or fire is always unique and is responsible for all biotransformation that takes place. Since energy can neither be created nor destroyed, Agni offers all the energy required for necessary bodily functions and activities. This energy is obtained from the nourishment we consume and the air we breathe. All the biological systems present within the body constantly work to transform this energy into a source that can be easily utilized by it. According to kaya chikitsa, there are six stages through which diseases develop. These stages are aggravation, accumulation, overflow, relocation, buildup, and manifestation of symptoms. An important treatment prescribed by kaya chikitsa is panchakarma, or body purification and cleansing. Purifying or cleansing your body helps rebalance all the doshas and bring them to a state of harmony. You will learn more about panchakarma in these chapters.

The most critical aspect of Kaya chikitsa is Agni or the digestive fire. This is important for your body's metabolism. Any imbalance in the internal Agni or fire of the digestive system results in general ailments. Agni helps convert food into body elements to promote your health.

Bala Chikitsa

Bala chikitsa is also known as kaumarabhritya. Bala means infants. This branch of Ayurveda deals with diseases of infants or pediatrics. Bala chikitsa, according to Acharya Sushruta, is associated with diseases or illnesses of children, the desirable qualities of a wet nurse, and anything that causes improper nourishment from breast milk. It also offers suggestions and practical tips to improve breast milk quality and the influence of grahas on a child's health. Antenatal care and puerperium management are also included in Bala chikitsa.

This branch of Ayurveda is associated with nurturing a child from conception to pregnancy and adolescence. The modern equivalence of this branch includes obstetrics and gynecology, and pediatrics. There are three aspects Bala chikitsa considers for treating children. The first consideration is that children are not fully equipped to express or explain any complaints they have. The second one is the dosage of medicine given to them is quite different, and the third is that the medicines need to be palatable. Treating children differs greatly from treating adults, so a separate branch of medicine was created under Ayurveda to deal specifically with children.

Graha Chikitsa

Graha chikitsa is known as Bhuta Vaidya, the modern-day equivalent of psychiatry. As mentioned previously, Ayurveda not only deals with physical health, but with your mental, emotional, and spiritual wellbeing too. Any disease not caused by an imbalance of the three doshas, and not falling into the categories mentioned above, comes under Graha chikitsa. It essentially refers to mental illnesses and disorders. There is no specific text associated with it, but most of the information about this branch of Ayurveda is obtained from

Atharva Veda and other sacred texts. Spiritual healing with Ayurveda is based on the concept of chanting a mantra or sound therapy. Mantras include specific combinations of consonants and vowels. The repetition of mantras is believed to cure several illnesses and Hindu and Buddhist religions.

This branch of Ayurveda deals with all sorts of mental diseases and their diagnosis and treatment. It offers advice on treating conditions such as epilepsy, insanity, or other disorders caused by an affliction of external factors. It also contains information to deal with conditions such as stress, depression, and insomnia.

Urdhwanga Chikitsa

All the areas above the clavicle, such as the eyes, nose, ears, mouth, teeth, throat, and head, are known as urdhwanga in Sanskrit. Urdhwanga chikitsa is a branch of Ayurveda equivalent to ophthalmology and otorhinolaryngology. Also known as shalakya tantara because shalakya or "a probe" is a unique instrument for the nose, throat, and eyes. Various subbranches include ophthalmology, otology, laryngology, dentistry, oral health, and anything associated with the cranium. It deals with the diagnosis, prognosis, prevention, and treatment of all diseases above the clavicle are included in this chikitsa. Acharya Sushruta noted 72 eye diseases and the corresponding treatments besides the diseases associated with the ears, nose, and throat. This chikitsa refers to ENT and ophthalmology.

Shalya Tantra

Shalya chikitsa or salyatnatra is the Ayurvedic equivalent of modern-day surgery in medicine. Long before surgical methods were introduced in the west, they were a part of Ayurvedic treatment. Ancient texts of Ayurveda delve into detail about surgery and surgical procedures. Sushruta's treatise, known as Sushruta Samhita, propagated sophisticated surgical practices prevalent in ancient India. It deals with different orthopedic and surgical procedures. Whether it is the removal of exogenous or endogenous bodies, it is included in it.

Apart from this, shalya chikitsa offers information about diagnosing and managing inflammatory conditions using surgical instruments. It also offers insight into how to prepare and apply different cauterization methods. This is used only for illnesses or diseases that other medicines can't cure. It offers information about helpful practices used to manage conditions such as fractures, osteoporosis, osteoarthritis, dislocation of joints, and other anorectal diseases. What is surprising about this branch of Ayurveda is it elaborately describes various instruments used to perform surgeries, such as scissors, scalpels, and holders.

Damshtra Chikitsa

Damshtra chikitsa is also known as visha chikitsa. Its modern-day equivalent is toxicology. It essentially deals with the treatment of poison. Poisons can be derived from ores, animals, and even plants. This branch of Ayurveda offers information about symptoms and treatments of anything associated with poisons, including snake and scorpion bites. Besides this, it includes helpful information about air and water pollution, epidemics, and toxins derived from various exogenous sources. By offering a list of symptoms used to recognize the presence of a specific toxin to their antidotes, everything about toxicology is available within this branch of Ayurveda.

Vishavaidyas were believed to be specialists in toxicology, and the traditional practice of toxicology is still prevalent among them. During ancient times, the primary responsibility of vishavaidyas was to protect members of the Royal households from being poisoned.

Jara Chikitsa

Jara chikitsa is also known as Rasayana chikitsa. Its modern-day equivalent is related to science and medicine in the field of rejuvenation. It offers medications and methodologies to maintain or preserve your youth, prolong the lifespan, and strengthen your immunity. It also includes information about symptoms and potential treatments to deal with the aging process and its associated health problems. It includes helpful information about the different steps that can be followed to promote longevity and good health. This branch includes treatments and therapies that produce an increase in the lifespan of neurons.

Vajikara

The Sanskrit word vaji means horse, and Karana translates to follow. This branch of Ashtanga Ayurveda deals with reproductive medicines and aphrodisiacs. It includes treatments and therapies to increase and improve the quality of semen and virility in men. It is also responsible for the purification of male and female genitalia. An important aspect of Ayurvedic teaching is it considers sex to be one of the essential parts of human life. Sex is believed to improve your overall health, endurance and is needed for procreation. This branch of Ayurveda explains the art of producing healthy children to create a better society. It deals with various conditions such as infertility and any other issues associated with reproductive fluids.

Globalization is one of the leading reasons there seems to be renewed interest in the holistic approach of Ayurveda. Even though there are eight branches in Ayurveda, there are only two ways to use them all. They can be used either as a preventive measure or a curative treatment. Instead of concentrating only on modern medicine's curative aspects, Ayurveda favors the preventive aspect of medicine.

Chapter 4: Chakras and Ayurveda

Chakras are the centers of energy present in the body. Lately, chakras have become a part of common parlance, but the concept isn't new. The origin of chakras can be traced back to ancient India to the sacred texts on Hinduism. Chakras have always been used in the healing process. They are found not just in Indian tradition but even in traditions from around the world like Taoism, Sufism, and even the ancient Mayans believed in their power.

The Flow of Energy in the Body

Energy is present all around us. The entire universe is made of energy. This might remind you of any physics classes you attended during school. Are you wondering how this is possible? Matter is present everywhere, right from the small atoms that make molecules to the electrons and protons that constantly collide to create energy. This energy is present within and around us. This energy present in your body is known as subtle energy. In Sanskrit, this energy is known as sukshma sharira. The word sukshma means subtle, while sharira means body. So, when put together, subtle energy is the personal energy field present within your body. This energy flows through certain energy centers known as chakras.

There are seven major chakras and several minor chakras. Each of the major chakras corresponds with one of the major organ systems. Previously, you were introduced to the idea that our body composition depends on personal energy or dosha compositions. These doshas or energy is reminiscent of the energy given out by the chakras. These chakras regularly interact with various organ systems in the body to maintain your overall health. Unless you learn to keep these chakras well balanced and spinning correctly, maintaining your health becomes difficult. Learning about these chakras helps increase your understanding of the energy concepts associated with Ayurveda.

The Root Chakra

The first chakra is the root chakra, commonly known as the base chakra. It is called the Muladhara chakra in Sanskrit and at the base of your spine. This chakra is between your anus and genitals. This chakra generates your survival instincts, and it is also related to the adrenaline glands that produce adrenaline. You can understand the gravity of any situation, and it will help you take a stand for yourself. Once your root chakra is balanced, you will be more confident than you used to be. The color associated with this chakra is red.

The Sacral Chakra

The Sanskrit name of the sacral chakra is the Svadhishthana chakra. This chakra is the second chakra, and is near your navel. The Sacral chakra is associated with the spleen and is usually found within two inches below the navel. This chakra strongly connects with the root or the base chakra. It also lets you determine your self-worth and discover your creative talents. This chakra generates confidence and the motivation to perform better, and any imbalances in this chakra would make you doubt yourself. Orange is the color associated with this chakra.

The Solar Plexus Chakra

The solar chakra is also known as Manipura. This chakra at the base of your sternum, near your solar plexus. Love springs from this place, and this chakra decides whether you love someone. Most of your emotions are also determined by the solar plexus chakra, like anger, passion, and the desire to become something better. You will have better control over your emotions if this chakra is well balanced, and you will learn how to trust yourself. Yellow is the color associated with this chakra.

The Heart Chakra

The heart chakra is also known as Anahata chakra in Sanskrit. This chakra is behind the breastbone, and the area surrounding the shoulder blades is included in it. This chakra commands spirituality and love - your mind and spirit are connected as one here. You will feel paranoid, unworthy, and lose your self-confidence when this chakra isn't balanced, and you will feel compassionate, friendly, and loving when it is well balanced. Green is the color associated with this chakra.

The Throat Chakra

The throat chakra is known as the Vishuddha chakra in Sanskrit. The fifth chakra is in your neck region, right around the collarbone. This chakra influences your ability to communicate and your speech and is considered the first of the three spiritual chakras. You may feel timid and quiet when the energy from this chakra is imbalanced and confident when balanced. Blue is the color associated with this chakra.

The Third Eye Chakra

The 3rd eye chakra is also known as Ajna chakra in Sanskrit. This chakra above the eyes and right in the middle of the forehead. According to Hindu mythology, Lord Shiva, also known as the destroyer, is one of the Trimurti. He is believed to have had a third eye, which is believed to trigger doomsday if ever opened. Your intuitive abilities and pure energy are located within this chakra. You will come across as egotistical and unfriendly when this chakra is unbalanced and optimistic, and self-confident when the sixth chakra is well balanced. Indigo is the color associated with this chakra.

The Crown Chakra

The Crown chakra is known as Sahasrara. This is the last chakra, and it is in your head, behind the skull. This is the center of spirituality and enlightenment. This chakra fuels your ability to stay energetic and your dynamic nature and, once you have balanced this chakra, it is safe to say that you have balanced all seven chakras. Violet is the color associated with this chakra.

The Pancha mahabuta principle was modified by ancient seers, which resulted in creating the Tri dosha theory. Doshas made it easier to understand and manage various diseases that the human body and mind suffer from. Sarpanch Maha bhuta principle is a structural classification of elements and the surrounding environment, while the Tri dosha explains functional aspects of the matrix. Ayurveda is based on this tridosha principle.

Energy can neither be created nor destroyed; it can only be transformed. This is one of the basic principles of science. This concept applies to the teachings of Ayurveda and the chakra system. The chakras are energy centers present in the body, each of which is associated with a specific organ function. When these chakras are spinning vibrantly and their energy is well balanced, it results in your overall wellbeing.

As mentioned earlier, each chakra is associated with a specific color, element, and even sounds. For instance, the bija mantras or the seed mantras used to balance the five lower chakras are associated with the Pancha mahabuta. Each of these sounds helps balance the energy of the chakras. Let's look at the relationship between bija mantras, elements, and their corresponding chakras.

The bija mantra for Muladhara chakra is LAM, and it is associated with Prithvi. The bija mantra for Svadhishthana chakra is VAM, and it is associated with jal. The bija mantra for Manipura chakra is RAM, and it is associated with Agni. The bija mantra for Vishuddha chakra is HAM, and it is associated with Akash. The colors of the chakras are also associated with different elements. For instance, yellow is associated with Prithvi, silver with jal, red with Agni, green with Vayu, and blue with Akash.

If you carefully go through the information, you'll discover that each chakra is associated with a specific element and color. This is the primary link between Ayurvedic philosophies and chakras. Understanding all this makes it easier to heal your body, mind, and soul using Ayurvedic teachings.

Chapter 5: The Ayurvedic Diet

Ayurveda offers a holistic approach to medicine that promotes the internal balance between your body, mind, and spirit. Five elements make up the universe, and these elements create the three doshas or the energies that circulate within everyone. The physiological functions differ from one dosha to another. For instance, your hunger, body temperature, and thirst are regulated by Pitta dosha, while Vata maintains the balance of electrolytes and your movement. But Kapha dosha is associated with joint function. In the previous chapters, understanding your dosha is important for improving your overall health and wellbeing. Determining your energy constitution helps create a diet that concentrates on specific foods that promote balance in all three doshas. The Ayurvedic diet is a vital part of Ayurveda and has been around for thousands of years.

An Ayurvedic diet helps create a diet plan that dictates guidelines based on what, how, and when you should eat according to your body type or dominant dosha. Here are the three doshas' primary characteristics that can determine which type is an ideal match for you.

The elements of Air and Space regulate Vata dosha. These individuals are extremely lively, full of energy, and highly creative. They have a light and thin body frame and struggle with anxiety, tiredness, and digestive troubles when their energy is not balanced.

Pitta dosha is regulated by fire and water energies. These individuals are hardworking, decisive, and intelligent and have a medium physical build, and are short-tempered. The common physical conditions they suffer from include heart disease, indigestion, and high blood pressure.

The elements of earth and water regulate the Kapha dosha. These individuals are loyal, well-grounded, and calm. They have a sturdier frame than the other doshas and gain weight easily. They also have a higher risk of developing depression, diabetes, and asthma.

Based on your dosha, the food you need to eat will differ. The Ayurvedic diet concentrates on this. By following an Ayurvedic diet, you can increase your internal balance, which improves your overall wellbeing. For instance, those with Pitta dosha should increase the consumption of energizing foods and have a cooling effect while limiting their intake of seeds, nuts, and all spices. Vata dosha will benefit from foods with a grounding and warm effect while limiting the intake of raw vegetables, dry fruits, and all bitter herbs. The Kapha dosha benefits from a diet rich in fresh fruits, vegetables, and legumes while limiting the intake of heavy and oily foods. Regardless of the dosha, an Ayurvedic diet restricts or eliminates processed foods, red meats, and all artificial sweeteners.

Benefits of an Ayurvedic Diet

Increased Intake of Whole Foods

Even though the Ayurvedic diet offers specific dietary guidelines for different doshas, the diet is generally rich in whole and fresh plant-based foods such as fruit, vegetables, legumes, and grains. By increasing your intake of such foods, your overall health will improve.

If you feed your body all the essential nutrients it needs, its general function will improve. It also reduces your intake of calorie-rich and nutrient-lacking processed foods devoid of dietary fiber, minerals, and nutrients. According to a study conducted by Bernard Srour et al. (2019), there is a direct link between processed foods and the risk of cardiovascular disorders. Processed foods also increase the risk of certain forms of cancer, according to the research conducted by Thibault Fiolet et al. (2018); since an Ayurvedic diet decreases the intake of these undesirable foods and replaces them with healthier ingredients, the risk of disease and metabolic disorders decreases.

Facilitates Weight Loss

According to a study conducted by Shikha Sharma et al. (2009), an Ayurvedic diet can increase the potential for weight loss. This study observed the weight loss progress of 200 participants with Pitta or Kapha doshas while following an Ayurvedic diet. The participants followed an Ayurvedic diet for three months and showed significant weight loss. Another study conducted by Jennifer Rioux et al. (2014) showed an average weight loss of 13 lbs. over nine months in participants who followed an Ayurvedic lifestyle. An Ayurvedic lifestyle combines an Ayurvedic diet and exercises. If weight loss is your priority, shifting to an Ayurvedic diet is a better approach.

Teaches Mindfulness

Mindfulness is an important aspect of all Ayurvedic teachings. Mindfulness is the ability to live in the moment without getting caught up with past or future worries. You do have the moment right now. There is no point worrying about things you can't change or control. By living in the moment, you become more aware of yourself and everything going on within and around you. You learn to pay close attention to how you feel. This results in increased self-awareness. Learn to eat mindfully. It means you need to pay attention to every morsel you consume. By doing this, you can understand the feelings of hunger and satiety. Instead of engaging in mindless eating, which almost always leads to overeating, mindfulness comes in handy. It makes you more conscious of what and how much you eat and the reasons for the same. It also increases your self-control.

Diet According to the Doshas

It has been repeatedly mentioned that you need to eat according to your doshas. This means that the foods you eat can help rebalance the dosha energy to improve your overall sense of wellbeing and health. Since the physical qualities of food affect your body's functioning, paying attention to what you eat or don't eat is important. In this section, let's look at a detailed eating guide for the three doshas.

Vata Dosha

To rebalance Vata energy, consume small portions of poultry, tofu, and seafood. The Vata energy benefits from cooked vegetables such as carrots, beets, sweet potatoes, green beans, onions, turnips, and radishes. Add plenty of fresh, sweet, and ripe fruit such as blueberries, strawberries, mangoes, plums, peaches, grapefruit, and bananas. Add dairy products such as yogurt, cheese, ghee, butter, and milk to your diet. You can consume various legumes and grains, including mung beans, all types of lentils, chickpeas, rice, and oats. You can include all types of nuts and seeds such as almonds, walnuts, pistachios, flax seeds, sunflower seeds, and chia seeds. Herbs and spices that are helpful for this dosha are cardamoms, ginger, basil, cloves, black pepper, cumin, and oregano.

Those with predominant Vata dosha should avoid red meat and light, dried, unripe fruit. Raw and cooked vegetables, including potatoes, cauliflower, broccoli, cabbage, mushroom, and tomatoes, are not ideal for this dosha. Many beans, including kidney beans, black beans, and Navy beans, along with certain grains like barley, rye, corn, wheat, millet, and buckwheat, are not suited for Vata dosha energy. Stay away from all bitter herbs such as thyme, coriander seeds, and parsley.

Pitta Dosha

Consume more dairy products such as ghee, butter, and milk, while consuming moderate amounts of protein, especially egg whites and tofu. Increase your intake of fresh and sweet fruit such as orange, pineapple, banana, pear, mango, and all types of melons. Sweet and bitter vegetables such as cauliflower, cabbage, bitter gourd, celery, cucumber, cabbage, zucchini, Brussels sprouts, sweet potato, and squash can rebalance Pitta energy. You can add various grains and legumes to your diet, including chickpeas, lentils, lima beans, kidney beans, mung beans, black beans, rice, wheat, oats, and barley. Add small amounts of nuts and seeds such as pumpkin seeds, sunflower seeds, flax seeds, and coconuts to your daily meals. Consume small amounts of healing spices such as turmeric, dill, cumin, cinnamon, cilantro, and black pepper.

Those with a predominant Pitta dosha need to avoid specific proteins such as egg yolks, seafood, and all types of red meats. They should also avoid acidic dairy products such as sour cream, buttermilk, and cheese. Apart from this, they need to stay away from all sour and unripe fruit and vegetables, including grapes, papaya, apricot, cherries, grapefruit, beets, tomatoes, onions, eggplant, and all types of peppers. Various grains they need to avoid are brown rice, rye, corn, and millets. They need to stay away from the herbs and spices that weren't included in the list mentioned above. Some nuts and seeds not suited for Pitta dosha are pine nuts, sesame seeds, walnuts, cashews, almonds, pistachios, and peanuts.

Kapha Dosha

To rebalance the Kapha energy present in your body, you need to consume small portions of protein-rich foods such as seafood and egg whites. Instead of full-fat dairy products, choose skimmed milk, soymilk, and goat's milk. You can add a variety of fresh fruits such as blueberries, pomegranates, cherries, apples, and dried fruits such as figs and prunes. You can also add raisins to your diet. Increase your intake of different healthy vegetables and legumes such as asparagus, onions, mushrooms, okra, radishes, potatoes, all green leafy vegetables and black beans, lentils, navy beans, and chickpeas. These ingredients are rich in dietary fiber and complex carbs that help improve your health and internal functioning. Different types of grains you can add to your diet are millet, corn, barley, buckwheat, oats, and rye. Consuming small amounts of pumpkin seeds, sunflower seeds, and flax seeds also help rebalance this dosha's energy. Apart from this, the Kapha energy benefits from many herbs and spices such as black pepper, turmeric, oregano, basil, cinnamon, ginger, cumin, and so on.

To rebalance the Kapha energy in your body, stay away from egg yolks, all types of red meats, and shrimp. Certain fruits and vegetables such as bananas, coconuts, figs, tomatoes, and mangoes and sweet potatoes, zucchini, and cucumbers, respectively, can harm Kapha's energy balance. Different legumes and grains you need to avoid include soybeans, kidney beans, miso, rice, all types of cooked cereals, and wheat. Cashews, brazil nuts, sesame seeds, walnuts, pecans, and pine nuts should be avoided while rebalancing your Kapha energy.

Depending on your type of dosha, you need to increase or decrease your intake of certain foods. Unless you become mindful of your food choices, improving your health becomes difficult. Since the energy obtained from foods directly regulates the doshas present within, an Ayurvedic diet will come in handy. Depending on the type of dosha that's predominant in your body, the Ayurvedic diet guidelines will differ.

Tips to Follow This Diet

Hundreds of years ago, Hippocrates said, "let food be your medicine." The principles of Ayurveda define the same philosophy. The Ayurvedic diet helps reestablish the balance between body and mind to enhance your overall sense of wellbeing and health. The various protocols determined by Ayurveda include suggestions about food selection, the timing of meals, and the state of awareness of your body and mind during these meals. All these factors either increase your vitality or toxicity. Vitality is known as Ojas and toxicity as ama. By following the Ayurvedic diet, you can increase your overall health and vitality while enhancing your energy levels through the food choices you consume. In the previous section, you were introduced to different foods ideal for the three doshas. Now, let us look at simple tips you can follow to incorporate an Ayurvedic style of eating.

Select the Right Foods

Ayurveda places immense importance upon the unique mind-body constitution of each person. This constitution is known as dosha. Any imbalance in dosha is known as vikruti, and it is usually a combination of two elements at high levels within an individual's physiology. By determining the right foods that reduce the heightened activity of the elements, harmony can be reestablished. You can use Ayurvedic principles to select and prepare foods ideal for your dosha type.

The elements of Air and Space govern the water dosha. It is naturally dry, light, cold, and rough. By consuming foods that counteract their basic characteristics, you can create harmony within your body. To restore balance and reduce excess levels of Vata dosha in your body, choose foods that are warm, hydrating, and rich in healthy fats, and with a grounding effect. But Pitta dosha is regulated by the elements of fire and water. This energy is naturally hot, sharp, or light, so you need to choose foods that cool your body down internally, have astringent properties, are mild, and minimize the fiery flames of pitta dosha.

Similarly, the Kapha dosha is governed by the elements of earth and water. The energy given out by this dosha is heavy, oil smooth, and cold. By consuming light, dry, rough, and warm foods, you can rebalance the energy of Kapha.

Unless you follow these simple protocols while selecting foods and their cooking methods, you can't rebalance your body's tridosha balance. Without this harmony, you can't improve your overall health and wellbeing.

Avoid Mindless Snacking

Whenever you consume a meal, Ayurveda suggests that your body goes through 3 stages of digestion. Unless these stages are complete, the buildup of ama or toxins increases. Supposing anything interrupts the digestive cycle, this creates incomplete digestion, of course. The simplest way to avoid incomplete digestion is by avoiding mindless snacking. Most of us are guilty of continually snacking throughout the day, regardless of our appetite.

Here is a basic understanding of the three stages of digestion your body goes through after a meal. Kapha energy is dominant during the first hour after consuming a full meal. You tend to feel heavy, full, and even drowsy during this period. The Pitta dosha elements govern the digestive process 2-4 hours after a meal. The production of hydrochloric acid increases within this stage, and your body's internal temperature increases. This internal temperature triggers your metabolism, where the meal is transformed into the energy your body requires. The Vata energy increases 4-5 hours after consumption of a meal. Toward the end of the digestive process, your body feels lighter, and space previously taken up by food is now free, so your hunger increases.

If you don't allow your body to complete this digestion cycle, which takes about five hours, the risk of indigestion increases. Incomplete digestion over a prolonged period results in the accumulation of ama. Accumulation of toxins in the body presents several symptoms that can be mild and moderate, or even excessive. This is one reason Ayurveda suggests that a healthy individual needs only three meals a day with no snacks between these meals. By doing this, you reduce the stress on the digestive system while ensuring your stomach functions optimally. When your digestive system functions optimally, your body gets all the nutrients and energy it needs to function as intended.

Eat Until You Are Satisfied

Every vehicle has a gas gauge that lets you determine whether or not it has sufficient fuel. If you think of your body as a vehicle, your stomach would be the gas gauge. Imagine it has numbers from 1 to 10 where number 1 determines it is empty and 10 denotes it is full. It is normal to want to eat when the gauge is around 2, while at 7, you will want to stop. If you eat before the gauge hits a 2 or eat past 7, it interrupts the digestive process. When you eat more than your stomach needs, most of your body's energies from the important physiological processes required to optimize your overall health are directed toward the digestive system.

When you eat more than what your body needs, it results in weight gain. Constant overeating increases the production of free radicals in the body, which trigger inflammation. Inflammation is also associated with speeding up the aging process, so learn to differentiate between actual hunger and mindless eating. Apart from this, become conscious of how much and when you eat. Make it a point to eat until you are full, and your hunger is satiated, but you are not overstuffed. If you constantly overstuff your body, it increases the stress on the digestive process. It also means your body starts hoarding unnecessary calories that are never fully utilized. By following the Ayurvedic diet, you consume only three meals a day and become more mindful of the food choices you make. By filling up on foods dense in nutrients, your body gets all the nourishment it needs. By avoiding mindless snacking, your calorie consumption reduces, and your body gets to utilize all the stored calories. Combining all these factors helps improve your overall health and derive the benefits associated with an Ayurvedic style of eating.

Consume Wholesome Foods

Prana is the life force and its presence in all the food you consume. Prana nourishes your body and giving it energy. It requires maintaining its overall health, energy, and vitality. The Pranic or energetic imprint of the food you consume is determined by various elements present in it, such as minerals, vitamins, and other phytonutrients. According to the Ayurvedic philosophy, the simplest way to increase your Ojas or vitality is by increasing prana. The most straightforward source of rich foods and prana are derived from the earth. Since their energy combines different natural elements such as water, sunshine, and the earth's energy, they are rich in prana. This is one reason why the Ayurvedic diet is rich and plant-based foods. By increasing your intake of fresh and wholesome ingredients, you are offering all the nutrients your body needs to function effectively and efficiently. While following an Ayurvedic diet, you need to reduce your consumption of processed and prepackaged foods and replace them with fresh ingredients. If you go through the dosha best food list discussed in the previous section, you will realize most of the food suggested fits the criteria mentioned above.

Pay Attention to The Six Tastes

According to Ayurveda, there are six tastes: sweet, sour, salty, bitter, pungent, and astringent. Every meal you consume needs to be a combination of all these tastes. Each taste is a combination of varying energies essential for maintaining your overall physiological functioning and health. When you incorporate all these into every meal, your body gets all the energy required to function effectively. Here are the different energetic properties associated with each of the six tastes. Sweet has a strengthening, grounding, and nourishing energy, while sour purifies and cleanses your body.

Similarly, salty foods regulate and balance your internal functioning, while bitter foods help detoxification and mineralization processes. Astringent foods are anti-inflammatory and have a cooling effect, while pungent ones stimulate and warm your body from the inside. It is easy to incorporate these tastes into every meal. For instance, by adding a pinch of salt, citrus, and spices, the energetic palate will be complete.

Be Aware of Your Cold Food Consumption

Inner fire or Agni determines the digestive power of your body. Agni is like a blazing bonfire. When it functions ideally, it is neither too hot nor too cold. This ensures your body can digest the food you consume effectively. A well-balanced internal fire brings about a sense of harmony to your thoughts, emotions, and experiences. To keep stoking your inner fire, you need to avoid foods that reduce its intensity. The simplest way to do this is by reducing your consumption of ice-cold beverages and foods. If you continuously consume all sorts of cold foods and drinks, the Agni in your body reduces automatically. Those with high Vata and Kapha dosha levels need to increase the consumption of warm foods and beverages. While the Pitta dosha benefits from cold foods and beverages, it doesn't mean consuming frozen foods.

Practice Mindful Eating

Mindfulness is a simple practice of staying engaged now without allowing your mind to get distracted by other thoughts. Mindful eating essentially means you are concentrating only on the meal you consume and nothing else. Most of us tend to read, watch TV, or do something else while eating. Ayurveda suggests that mealtime is a brilliant opportunity that allows you to connect with the inherent energy associated with the foods you consume. Learn to pay attention to the color, taste, flavor, and texture of the food you eat. Savor every bite, chew carefully, and swallow. Practicing mindful eating avoids the risk of overeating and ensures that you know your body signs of hunger and satiety.

The Gap Between Meals and Bedtime

Sleep is considered healing and restorative. While you are sleeping, most of your body's energy is diverted from physiological processes such as digestion and redirecting internal repairs and healing. Your body gets to heal, restore and repair itself while the mind gets to process all the thoughts, emotions, feelings, and experiences of the day you had. This is one reason Ayurvedic practices suggest you need to give your body a break before bedtime. Ideally, avoid eating at least three hours before bedtime. The last meal of the day you consume needs to be light, ensuring most of the digestive process is completed before you go to sleep. When your body's internal energy is free during deep slumber, its internal repair and healing mechanisms work as intended.

Drink Herbal Teas

You need to stoke the internal fire or Agni to ensure the digestive system's health and functioning. A great way to do this is by sipping on hot herbal teas between the meals. Drinking herbal teas can also rebalance the energy of different doshas. Another benefit of drinking herbal teas is it helps keep hunger pangs at bay and reduce the urge to snack. Herbal teas not only stoke the digestive Agni but help with detoxification too. Pitta energy can benefit from teas that are hot or cold made with herbs such as coriander, rose, and peppermint. Vata dosha benefits from herbs with a calming and grounding effect, such as cloves, cinnamon, and ginger. The Kapha dosha helps with digestion and destabilization of your energy and benefits from teas made of black pepper, cardamom, and licorice.

Make Lunch the Largest Meal

Your body's Agni is potent when the sun is at its highest position, so consume the largest meal of the day at lunch. Have a light breakfast and dinner while consuming a massive meal at lunch. This ensures your body has more energy to digest even heavy and difficult-to-digest foods effectively. It also gives your body plenty of energy needed to get through the rest of the day.

By following the simple tips and suggestions in this section, you can reap all the benefits of the Ayurvedic diet. Whether you want to improve your health or lose weight, there is a lot to gain from this diet.

Note: If you have any preexisting health conditions such as diabetes or high blood pressure, always consult your healthcare provider before making any dietary changes.

Chapter 6: Meditation in Ayurveda

We live in a world where our senses are in constant overdrive due to all the stimulation we are exposed to. Meditation offers a respite from all this chaos, which guides our lives towards peace. Practicing meditation is like training a specific muscle in your body. This is not something you can achieve overnight, but with mindful practice and a little effort, you can get the hang of it. Meditation is all about tapping into your inner stillness and self-reflection. It allows you to block unnecessary feelings and emotions without becoming judgmental. By observing all that you feel and think, you get a better sense of what you are feeling and the reasons for those feelings. Once you understand this, controlling and regulating your feelings and emotions becomes easier. Since your emotions are responsible for your thoughts, and your thoughts determine your actions and behaviors, regulating your thoughts is vital. Meditation allows you to live in the moment without worrying about the past or the future. It increases your sense of self-awareness. This self-awareness is not just about your physical body, but your mental and emotional self too. It allows you to connect with your inner self while harmonizing the relationship between your body, mind, and spirit.

Benefits of Meditation

Meditation is a conscious process of training your mind to concentrate and regulate all the thoughts you think. It not only increases your self-awareness but makes you more aware of your surroundings too. It is also a great way to reduce any stress you experience while enhancing your concentration. This is one of the best ways to create a positive outlook toward life while working on self-discipline and forming healthy lifestyle habits. In this section, let's look at all the different benefits associated with meditation.

Stress Reduction

One of the most common reasons people turn to meditation is because of its stress-reducing capabilities. Whether it is physical or mental stress, it is caused by a stress-inducing hormone known as cortisol. Excess production of cortisol prevents you from getting good quality sleep at night, increases your blood pressure, increases the risk of anxiety and depression, and results in fatigue. Mindful meditation increases your ability to deal with stress effectively without letting it govern your life. While meditating, you are essentially teaching your mind to focus only on the moment and not worrying about the past or future. When you live in the moment, it becomes easier to concentrate on all that you are doing. This is a great way to reduce stress. It also increases your productivity.

Regulates Anxiety

When stress levels reduce, anxiety also reduces automatically. According to a meta-analysis conducted by David W Orme-Johnson et al. (2014), meditation helps reduce anxiety levels. In another study conducted by Elizabeth A. Hoge et al. (2014), meditation helps reduce anxiety and manage its symptoms in those with a generalized anxiety disorder. When you train your mind to concentrate only on a specific thought without getting overwhelmed by everything that's happening, has happened, or might happen, the chances of getting overwhelmed reduce. By thinking clearly and calmly, you are reducing any anxiety you experience. Clear thinking is also crucial for better decision-making.

Better Emotional Health

Meditation is believed to improve your self-image and help develop a positive outlook toward life in general. In a systematic review and meta-analysis conducted by Madhav Goyal et al. (2014), the symptoms of depression improved in 3500 adults when they were practicing meditation. Meditation helps regulate your thoughts and understand your responses. Instead of merely reacting to everything that happens in your life, meditation promotes logical responses. When you understand and learn of negative thoughts and feelings you experience, replacing them with positive behaviors and thoughts becomes more effortless. Meditation promotes self-awareness, and this is how it reduces the scope of negativity in your life. Whenever you are stressed, your body's cytokines or inflammatory chemicals are produced in response to that stress. This can negatively affect your overall mood and result in depression. According to a study conducted by Eshvendar Reddy Kasala et al. (2014), meditation reduces the risk of depression by reducing inflammatory chemicals within the body.

Promotes Self-Awareness

Meditation is believed to enhance self-awareness vital for self-development; during meditation, you have an opportunity for self-inquiry and self-introspection. You get a better understanding of yourself and how you relate to everything else in your life and others around you. It gives you the required tools to recognize harmful thoughts or self-defeating thought patterns. By increasing your awareness of all this, it becomes easier to develop positive and constructive patterns instead of dwelling on the self-defeating ones.

Better Attention Span

When you meditate, you learn to increase your attention span without getting overwhelmed by everything else that happens in your life. Most of us are guilty of multitasking. Whenever you multitask, you are essentially distributing your limited attention to multiple things. It might sound like a good idea because many believe it increases their productivity, but it is not valid. Multitasking merely reduces your focus and overall productivity. When you meditate, you are fine-tuning your attention span and increasing its overall strength. Even meditating for as little as 13 minutes daily can increase your attention, memory, promote emotional regulation, and shift your overall mood for the better. All this was obtained from a study conducted by Julia C Basso et al. (2019).

Promote Positive Feelings

Meditation is believed to increase positive feelings, not just toward the self and the practitioner's life but also to others. According to a meta-analysis conducted by Julieta Galante et al. (2014), meditation increases feelings of compassion toward oneself and others. Meditation promotes kindness. Your thoughts regulate your actions. When you think and feel good about yourself, it shows in your actions.

Meditation is a relaxation technique that helps calm your mind and give it the rest it needs to increase your state of awareness. It enables you to get a better understanding of yourself and connect with your center of consciousness. It is not a religious practice, but it can be used to increase your spirituality. While you're meditating, your mind becomes calm, quiet, and focused. Even while you are awake and alert during a meditation session, your mind does not concentrate on things around you. Instead, its focus shifts inward. Instead of worrying about the external world, it explains the world present within you.

Most of us are conditioned to examine our external words from a young age. In our bid to do this, we often forget about the world that exists within us. Unfortunately, most of us aren't aware of our true selves and are not in contact with it. All this confusion and disappointment we experience often stems from a lack of self-understanding. The human mind has a conscious and subconscious portion. The subconscious controls a variety of functions performed by the mind. It stores your memories, dreams, and even regulating sleep. The conscious mind is easy to control, but the subconscious isn't. Meditation helps you gain control over this part of your mind.

Meditation is a brilliant technique that helps discipline your mind while resisting the urge to give in to all distractions we surround ourselves with. Learning to control your thoughts and overcome distractions becomes easier with meditation. Meditation helps calm your mind, fine-tune your focus, offers a better sense of clarity, strengthens your communication, and relaxes your body and mind. During meditation, your body undergoes physiological changes. It is believed to reduce your blood sugar levels and blood pressure too. When your blood pressure levels are well within control, your anxiety and stress levels reduce automatically.

Stress is a leading cause of chronic pain and several illnesses. By tackling stress, you can overcome the problems associated with it, such as headaches, digestive troubles, and even insomnia. Meditation can improve the health of your immune system and increase your energy levels. Besides reducing anxiety and improving your mood, meditation results in improved mental and emotional stability. It helps fine-tune your focus while working on strengthening your intuition. Meditation increases your self-awareness. So, next time you feel overwhelmed or anxious, take a break and meditate. When you are calmer, your ability to make better decisions increases automatically. Better decisions mean positive actions. Meditation is the key to creating a life you desire free from all forms of stress.

How to Meditate

The practice of meditation differs from one person to another, but meditation's primary objective always stays the same. It's about achieving a sense of contentment while harmonizing your body, mind, and spirit. Meditation is defined as the continuous flow of thought or perception. It is the simplest way to achieve self-awareness while bringing about a sense of natural order and harmony into your life through constant observation. It gives you a chance to tap into your inner self and discover the tranquility or peace present within. It is a healing practice that increases your sense of relaxation and promotes inner calm. Ayurveda prescribes meditation under Daivavyaprashaya chikitsa.

Meditation is important for everyone, and we all benefit from it. It brings about a sense of balance in your life, which is vital in this chaotic world. Since Ayurveda concentrates on creating therapies and relaxation techniques based on an individual's Prakriti, the meditation practices suggested by it vary. There are different meditation available for varying Prakriti. Your Prakriti depends on your state of mind, the state of sattva, tamas, or rajas.

Our Prakriti depends on the different dosha constitutions within the body. For instance, the Kapha mind always desires to be engaged in work while Vata should be still and calm. Selecting an appropriate meditative technique is based on your internal Prakriti or mental constitution and your state. The simplest way to rebalance and strengthen the harmony between mind and body is by meditating according to your Prakriti, following an Ayurvedic diet, and eliminating all activities which overwhelm your senses.

The energy of Vata and rajas are similar since they are associated with movement and irregularity. Pranayama works to stabilize your Vata mind. Pranayama is a practice of mindful breathing. Kapha minds are slow and usually need to be kick-started. Any meditative practice that engages the Kapha mind is helpful. Dwelling on contemplative questions and guided visualization are ideal meditative practices for Kapha doshas. Another technique you can use is walking meditation. This technique's primary idea is to engage the Kapha energy and keep it busy to prevent it from slowing down. But Pitta minds need to be quiet and calm. Pranayama works brilliantly well for this energy that needs to be cooled and calmed. You will learn more about meditative techniques ideal for different doshas in the next section. For now, let's look at simple tips you need to remember while practicing meditation.

Meditation is an exercise in mindfulness. The simplest way to make the most of any exercise routine is consistency. Make it a point to practice meditation at a specific time daily. The more you practice, the more adept you become at regulating your thoughts and mind. Practice meditation in a specific place and at a specific time.

The best time to meditate is early in the morning. Practice meditation for around 5- 15 minutes when you wake up in the morning. At this point, your mind is not clouded with thoughts or worries. It is free from the clutter of daily life.

Whenever you are meditating, make sure that you are facing either East or North. These directions are believed to be ideal for meditation. While meditating, sit with your back straight, and ensure that your neck and head are aligned. Don't stiffen your muscles but instead, keep your body loose. By relaxing your body physically, it becomes easier to relax your mind.

While meditating, try to keep your mind calm. Don't force yourself to concentrate on any specific thoughts. Instead, allow your thoughts to come and go. Don't get fixated on the idea of forced relaxation. While your thoughts are passing by, don't judge them. Permit yourself to let your mind run free.

Regulating your breathing is a great way to focus your mind and let go of mental clutter. To meditate, find a calm spot, and close your eyes. Concentrate on breathing in and out deeply for five minutes. Whenever your mind wanders, focus on your breath and redirect it to the present. Don't get bogged down by past or future worries. Instead, appreciate the moment available right now.

Allow your mind to wander wherever it wants to. After practicing deep breathing for a couple of minutes, slowly hone it toward a focal point of your choice. Ensure this is the only thing you think about throughout the meditation. You might not be able to do this initially. During the initial sessions of meditation, concentrate only on your breathing and nothing else. Notice how the air enters and exits your body. Concentrate on this flow of oxygen.

Meditation According to Doshas

Meditation helps eliminate mental clutter and shifts your focus to the goals that matter. By increasing your self-awareness and freeing up mental space, you can eliminate unhelpful thoughts and make more space for positivity. Meditation can help balance all three doshas. In the previous chapter, you were introduced to each of the three doshas' characteristics and now, let's look at meditative practices ideal for them.

Vata Meditation

The Vata energy is usually subtle, light, and constantly moving. These qualities can manifest themselves as worry, restlessness, anxiety, or even fears when left unchecked. Excess Vata energy can leave you feeling jittery and overactive. Whether it is excessive stress or unsettling changes, several reasons exist that can imbalance the Vata dosha. An ideal meditative practice for Vata energy is associated with mantra meditation. A mantra is usually a phrase rhythmically repeated to calm the mind and improve your focus. You can use mala beads. These are similar to rosary beads and can track the repetitions of the mantras you say. Since these beads are tangible, holding them in your hands ensures that your Vata energy is grounded in that moment. If you don't have mala beads or don't want to use them, you can always repeat the mantra for 5-15 minutes or until you feel calmer. Here are the simple steps you can follow to rebalance your Vata dosha using mantras.

You need to select a mantra that personally resonates with you. It can be a phrase or even a word. The language of the mantra doesn't matter. You can use any language you prefer. If you are confused about the phrase to use, choose a word. A simple word you can use is calm or peace. Here is a phrase that works well for Vata energy, and it is "yoga seizes the fluctuations of the mind." This quote is from Patanjali's second sutra.

Now that you have chosen a mantra or a phrase, sit comfortably and relax your hands. Keep your body loose and consciously soften your facial muscles. Ensure that your eyes are closed during the meditation. If you are using a mala, hold it in your right hand, so it is placed over your middle, ring, and little fingers.

Whenever you repeat the prayer or the mantra, move the mala beads one at a time. You can repeat this mantra out loud, whisper, or even repeat it mentally. This is up to you. You are essentially repeating the mantra once for every bead you move. Ensure that you fall into a soothing rhythm of repeating this mantra. You need to repeat it 108 times or until you feel calm and focused. Once you feel calm, slowly open your eyes and get on with your daily activities.

Pitta Dosha

Pitta dosha requires peace to counter its sharp and hot qualities. Excess stress or stimulation results in Pitta dosha losing its internal sense of peace and tranquility. Excess Pitta energy often manifests itself as impatience, anger, frustration, and a general feeling of irritation. By choosing a meditating technique that calms your mind, you can overcome its negative manifestations. The simplest way to stabilize the energy of Pitta dosha is through a simple breathing meditation. The intense energy of Pitta dosha can be redirected by using the breath as an anchor; this will keep you grounded during the meditation. Pitta dosha favors planning, organizing, and prioritizing different activities. By taking a break, you can concentrate on the essential and crucial aspects of life. Make a conscious effort to reset your mind and concentrate on rebalancing the Pitta energy. Here is a simple meditation exercise suitable for Pitta dosha.

To get started, find a comfortable and quiet spot for yourself. Ensure that the chosen spot is away from all distractions, and you will not be interrupted during the meditation. You need to sit comfortably. While sitting cross-legged, always keep your back straight, shoulders loose, and your hands should rest in your lap with the palms facing upward. Your body needs to be loose and fluid. If you tense your muscles, this tension follows into your meditation too.

Close your eyes and relax the muscles in the jaw and face. If you are thinking about how to do this, maintaining a neutral expression will help you achieve the goal.

In this meditation, the primary focus needs to be on your breathing. Concentrate only on the movement of your abdomen as you inhale and exhale. Don't try to regulate your breathing but, instead, merely observe the natural movement and how the breath feels within your body.

Continue this meditation for around 10- 20 minutes or until you feel calm and relaxed. It is quite simple to follow this meditation. It can be easily added to your busy schedule. You can perform this simple meditation any time, regardless of where you are. You need only to find a quiet spot for yourself, close your eyes, and shift all your attention to your breathing. Initially, you might struggle to do this, but eventually, you will get the hang of it. The other two doshas will benefit from this meditation exercise too.

Kapha Dosha

An ideal meditative practice for Kapha dosha is walking meditation. Excess Kapha energy manifests itself as sluggishness, lethargy, and foggy thinking. It also reduces your general motivation. To prevent the over-accumulation of Kapha energy, which is generally heavy, thick, and damp, you must learn to rebalance it. The best way to do this is by promoting movement and circulation to get through the sluggishness associated with Kapha dosha. Using a meditative technique with opposing qualities will leave you feeling lighter, livelier, and more energetic. Walking meditation will help eliminate stalled energy. It increases your mental clarity while giving your body the required motion to overcome the heavy and dampening qualities of Kapha dosha.

Here are the simple steps you can follow to practice walking meditation.

Set aside 15- 20 minutes daily to practice walking meditation. You can either practice it outside or indoors. If the weather conditions are favorable, try practicing walking meditation outdoors. By spending time in nature, you are naturally increasing your body's exposure to desirable natural elements. For walking meditation, it is always better to walk barefoot. Remove your shoes and socks and try to increase the sensation and stimulation for your feet. The next time you get started with this meditation, assume the mountain pose. Mountain pose is also known as tadasana in yoga. To get started, stand straight with your feet slightly apart. Ensure that your weight is equally balanced on your feet. Without hardening your lower abdomen, tighten the muscles in your thighs and gently push the knees out. Now, press your shoulders into the back while ensuring your crown directly aligns with your pelvis. Take a couple of deep breaths and pay attention to how you feel.

Start breathing naturally, keep your gaze downward, and walk slowly and rhythmically. You can walk in a circular path or a long line. While walking, pay attention to three words with each step you take. The three words are to lift, move, and place. Ensure that you concentrate on nothing else other than these three things. By focusing your mind's attention on the soles of your feet, you will feel grounded. Try to feel every movement you make. At the end of the meditation, stop moving and notice how you feel. By concentrating only on your movement, you are clearing your mental clutter while refocusing your attention on the present moment.

By following the meditation practices discussed in this chapter, you can regulate your mind while stabilizing the tridoshas. Meditation is a skill, and it takes consistent practice and effort. Don't be disappointed if you don't get the results you desire on the first try. Be patient, practice the meditation consistently, and it will get easier. You can experiment with different meditation exercises until you find one that suits your needs and requirements.

Chapter 7: Yoga Practice in Ayurveda

Yoga is a popular form of exercise across the world these days. It originated in India and then spread to all parts of the globe. Yoga and meditation are two practices that can improve your overall health and wellbeing while reestablishing the connection between your body, mind, and spirit. Yoga shares a close connection with the practice of Ayurveda. It is not a new concept, and understanding it increases awareness of your body and all that it needs.

What is Yoga?

Yoga is an ancient practice, and its history goes back to over 5000 years ago. It is based on ancient Indian philosophy, and when you hear the word yoga, the first thing that may pop into your head may be a couple of complex poses and positions. There is so much more to yoga than just that. Yoga combines physical postures, meditation or relaxation techniques, and breathing exercises. In recent times, yoga has become a popular form of physical exercise that helps enhance your control over the mind while improving your overall wellbeing.

Even though yoga enjoys a lengthy history, there's no written record of the creator of yoga. All the male and female yoga practitioners, known as yogis and yoginis, respectively, practiced and taught yoga even before yoga practices were recorded in the written word. The yogis and yoginis passed all their knowledge and information to their disciples. These disciples further spread the information they had about yoga and its wonderful benefits and healing abilities.

A 2000-year-old written record of yogic philosophy known as yoga sutra was written by Patanjali, an ancient Indian sage. This book is primarily a guide to master and gain complete control over your mind, emotions, and body to increase your spirituality. This is believed to be one of the earliest written records of yoga and one of the oldest texts in existence in the world. Patanjali's yoga sutra also offers the framework for all modern yoga practices prevalent today.

Even though postures and poses are popular in yoga, they were not a crucial part of India's original yogic traditions. Fitness was not the primary goal of yoga. Instead, the practitioners and followers of yoga often concentrated on increasing their spiritual awareness and energy, calming their mind, and concentrating on the breath to harmonize the relationship between the body, mind, and soul.

Prima facie, Ayurveda, and yoga might sound like two different philosophies. Once you learn these concepts, you will discover several similarities that make them complementary therapies. The most obvious similarity between these two practices is their Vedic roots. These practices were created to improve your overall sense of wellness and offer a holistic approach to health. They are derived from the same Vedic scriptures and have similar underlying principles and beliefs about holistic wellbeing and holistic approach to health. Yoga concentrates on harmonizing the connection between the body, mind, spirit, while Ayurveda focuses on stabilizing the tridoshas through positive dietary and lifestyle changes.

Combining Ayurveda and yoga can improve your overall sense of wellbeing. It allows you to become more aware of your body and promote natural healing. You are not only improving your health but also curing yourself by purging all toxins present within.

An important concept of Ayurveda is to thoroughly understand your body composition, doshas and make lifestyle changes according to what is best for your dosha. We are all unique, and our unique constitution is governed by our emotional and physical makeup, including any of our lifestyle patterns. Ayurveda works by prescribing specific changes and practices to help restore harmony between nature and all doshas in the body. Similarly, even yoga tries to create or establish this sense of harmony by a combination of yoga poses, breathing exercises, and meditation practices. When you do this, your body and mind are finally in synchronization. Meditative and breathing exercises are a great way to increase your spirituality while promoting internal healing.

Another important similarity between Ayurveda and yoga is that they focus on holistic health solutions customized according to your needs and requirements. Several yoga poses are ideal for each of the three doshas. Depending on the dosha you want to heal or balance, the yoga pose you choose will differ. This is pretty much the same philosophy followed in Ayurveda too. These techniques work by utilizing the healing power of nature and leveraging it to enhance your overall sense of wellbeing.

You can't discount that both these philosophies share a similar objective. Their goal is to help improve your health and assure that your energies are well balanced. It also ensures that your body, mind, senses, and soul are well balanced. When you put all this together, it automatically increases your overall sense of wellbeing. When there is harmony between these components, your life changes for the better.

The Benefits of Yoga

Your flexibility increases whenever you move and stretch your muscles. When you practice yoga regularly, your back, shoulder, hamstrings, and hip muscle flexibility increases. When this flexibility increases, any tension present then reduces. The lack of flexibility and excess tension in muscles reduces mobility. This immobility over a period increases the risk of chronic pain. With yoga, you can reverse this process. It's a popular misconception that yoga poses are extremely difficult and tricky to perform. Well, this is not true. Most yoga poses involve some form of stretching or other. All it takes is a little practice to develop the flexibility desired for complicated yoga poses. Also, yoga poses use your body weight in varying ways. For instance, you tend to support your body weight on one leg while performing a tree pose. Similarly, in the downward dog position, you use your arms to support the body weight. These are like regular body-weight exercises. You may not realize it, but these poses help increase your muscle strength and mobility.

Yoga poses help increase muscle strength, develop lean muscle, and improve body muscle tone without bulking up. If you like the idea of lean and strong muscles, perform yoga today. Another benefit of yoga is you can do these poses from the comfort of your living room. Don't go to a specific place to perform yoga.

Most of the yoga poses require some form of balance. Meditation helps balance your mind, while yoga brings with it a sense of stability to your body. It is also believed to increase your core strength. Most of the yoga poses require low-intensity movement. It means you can perform them without increasing the stress on your joints or muscles. Even individuals with arthritis can perform yoga without increasing stress on the joint or worsening their condition.

Most of us lead extremely hectic lives. A lot of us spend a significant portion of our day hunched in front of desktops and laptops, which leads to poor posture and increases the risk of low back problems. Even if you spend a lot of your time driving, you may notice certain tightness in your upper torso. This posture can cause spinal compression. You can use yoga to reverse this process. Lower back pain can be addressed with yoga poses, such as the cobra pose.

We breathe without even paying any conscious thought to it. Yoga is not just about physical poses but includes a variety of breathing exercises too. These breathing exercises are specifically designed to shift your attention to your breathing. For instance, pranayama encourages conscious breathing. When you learn to breathe correctly, your body obtains a steady flow of oxygen. When it receives all the oxygen it needs, it helps calm the nervous system and promote its internal functioning. Becoming conscious of how you breathe is also a meditative exercise.

By shifting all your attention to the yoga poses you perform, you are fine-tuning your focus. When you do this, your mind automatically calms down. Meditation and yoga always go hand in hand. By concentrating on your breathing, your focus moves away from all overwhelming thoughts running through your mind. When this happens, you automatically feel calmer and lighter. When your mind is calm, it becomes easier to disengage from negative thoughts.

The simplest way to let go of any stress you experience is by engaging in physical activities. Whenever your body concentrates on physical movement, the production of stress-inducing hormones slows down. It also releases hormones that counteract stress and elevate your mood, known as endorphins. By performing yoga, you are not only calming the mind but are increasing the levels of feel-good hormones within your body. To take a break from the daily stress you experience, perform yoga. Physical exercise also makes it easier to fall asleep at night. Your ability to sleep through the night decreases when you're body and mind are exhausted. Good quality of sleep makes you feel more energetic and refreshed. Since sleep is restorative and healing for your body, yoga promotes good sleep at night.

Yoga makes you more aware of your body. An important benefit of yoga is it strengthens the connection between your body, mind, and spirit. When these three elements are synchronized, your sense of health and overall wellbeing increase. That enables you to identify the subtle movements important for your overall health.

As mentioned earlier, depending on your dosha, the yoga poses you need to choose will differ. In this section, let's look at some simple and easy yoga poses you can follow for each of the three doshas.

Yoga Poses for Vata Dosha

Mountain Pose

The mountain pose is known as tadasana in Sanskrit. Learning the Sanskrit names of these poses may seem a little complicated, but it will enhance your overall understanding of yogic traditions. This posture is often used for grounding. To get started, stand up straight with your feet placed hip-width apart. Spread your feet apart slightly and ensure your weight is evenly distributed on both feet from front to back and the sides. Tighten the muscles in your thighs and raise your arms overhead while you inhale. Stretch your arms as high as you can, and your fingertips need to be aligned with the head. While you do this, slowly press down into your feet. Close your eyes and concentrate on taking long and slow breaths. Breathe in and out through your nose. There should be no strain or struggle while you hold onto this position. Breathe, relax, and note how you feel and let your body relax. Hold onto this pose for three minutes and slowly lower your arms to your side while you exhale.

Stand Forward Bend

This pose is known as Uttanasana in Sanskrit. To get started, stand straight with your feet placed hip-width apart. As you inhale, raise your arms and move your waist forward and lower your arms to the side. Your position should be such that your hands rest on your ankles or shins. Try to reach for your ankles, and if you can't, try to bend forward as much as you can while keeping your head and neck fully relaxed. Straighten your knees gently and let your hands move from the shins to rest on the floor if possible. If not, hold onto your ankles and keep your body relaxed. Close your eyes and concentrate on taking a long slow, and deep breath through your nose. You need to inhale and exhale through your nose. While you inhale, notice any tension or tightness you experience in the body. As you exhale, allow the tension to move away from the specific area and let yourself relax. Keep breathing slowly and deeply for 3 minutes. To release this position, you need to slowly move back to a standing position one vertebra at a time. Stand quietly for a couple of breaths before you end this pose.

Seated Spinal Twist

This pose is known as Ardha matsyendrasana. To get started, assume a sitting position and extend your legs. You can extend your left leg or bend it toward your buttock. Now, bend your right leg at the knee while your foot is placed facing outward from your left knee. Place your right hand behind your body, and keep it as close to your back as you can. You need to balance your weight on your right hand and use it as a kickstand to straighten your spine. Your left elbow needs to be hooked behind the right knee. Elongate your spine, inhale slowly, and exhale slowly. While you Excel, twist your torso to look over your right shoulder. Hold onto this position for 2 or 3 minutes while you take long and deep breaths. After this, change sides and repeat this on the other side.

Knees to Chest Pose

This pose is known as Apanasana. Find a comfortable surface and lie on your bark. Gently draw your knees inward toward your chest. Now, wrap your arms or hands around your legs and try to move your knees closer to the collarbone. While you do this, elongate your spine and do not raise your head off the floor. With your head on the floor, slowly move your chin toward your chest while your shoulders melt backward. Before you close your eyes, try to look at the space present between your knees and arms. Keep breathing slowly and deeply. Let your belly press against your thighs, which helps massage the internal organs. Hold onto this pose for three minutes and release slowly. While releasing this pose, slowly extend your legs until they are straight with your arms placed by your sides.

Legs Up the Wall

This pose is known as Viparita Karani. To get started with this position, move close to a wall such that your glutes are pressed against it. Slowly extend your legs until they form an "L" and are perpendicular to the floor while resting against the wall. Your calves, back of the thighs, and heels will rest on the wall. Flex your feet and let your arms rest by your side. Breathe in slowly and deeply while you close your eyes. Hold onto this position for 5- 10 minutes. To release this pose, roll onto your side while your knees are tucked. Hold onto this position for two minutes before you get up.

Yoga Poses for Pitta Dosha

Downward Facing Dog

This pose is known as adho mukha svanasana. It is believed to reduce any tension in your body and increases relaxation. To get started, get onto your hands and knees on a comfortable surface. Your hands should be placed directly under your shoulders and knees under the hips. Spread your hands as wide as you possibly can such that the index finger and thumb press into the mat or ground.

Your elbows will turn outward in this position. Lift your tailbone and glutes while lengthening your hamstrings. Your stomach must be as close to the thighs as possible while your ears are between your biceps and heels pressed toward the floor. Even if your heels don't touch the ground, don't worry because it takes a little practice. Keep breathing deeply and evenly while you relax into this position. Hold onto this pose for a minute and release it.

Head to Knee Pose

This pose is known as Janu sirsasana. To get started:

1. Get onto your hands and knees on a comfortable surface. Your hands should be placed directly under your shoulders and knees under the hips.

2. Spread your hands as wide as you can such that the index finger and thumb press into the mat or ground. Your elbows will turn outward in this position.

3. Lift your tailbone and glutes while lengthening your hamstrings. Your stomach must be as close to your thighs as possible while your ears are between your biceps and heels pressed toward the floor.

4. Even if your heels don't touch the ground, don't worry because it takes a little practice.

5. Keep breathing deeply and evenly while you relax into this position.

6. Hold onto this pose for a minute and release it.

Superman Pose

This pose is known as Viparita Salabhasana. To get started, lie on your stomach on the mat. Your limbs need to be on the floor while your legs and arms extend outward. As you inhale, lift both your arms and legs off the ground while balancing your weight on the lower abdominal muscles and pelvis. Hold on to this pose so you can breathe fully and comfortably, even in an elevated state. Relax your body and hold onto it for 2- 3 minutes.

Child's Pose

This pose is known as garba sona. To get started, assume a kneeling position on the floor and fold forward while your stomach rests on the thighs and forehead touches the ground. Your arms need to be fully extended in front of your body while you elongate the spinal cord. Your palms need to rest on the floor fully. Hold onto this pose for up to three minutes while you inhale and exhale slowly. To end the pose, press up on your hands and knees to shift onto your back.

Supine Spinal Twist

This pose is known as the supta matsyendrasana. To get started, lie on the floor on your back and lift your arms to the sides to form a "T." Gently bend your right knee and bring it closer to your chest across your body and onto the floor. Ensure that your right shoulder rests on the ground while your balance is maintained by your left hand. Your left hand ensures that your right knee stays down on the floor. Move your head to look over the right shoulder. Breathe in deeply through the nose. Feel the breath fill your hip, ribcage, shoulder, and armpit on the right side of your body. While you exhale, concentrate on relaxing any tension present in these areas. Hold onto this pose for 2-3 minutes on one side before shifting to the other. Once you complete this, lie down on your back and relax for ten minutes.

Yoga Poses for Kapha Dosha

The Tree Pose

This pose is known as Vrikasana. To get started:

1. Stand with your feet placed hip-width apart.

2. Shift your body's entire weight onto the right foot and ensure that your foot stays firmly connected with the floor at all times.

3. Gently move the left foot up to be placed right below the right knee while you press back the left knee as if touching an imaginary wall behind.

4. Find a spot on the floor in front of you and concentrate on it.

5. While you inhale, raise your arms overhead and keep them straight.

6. Hold on to this pose and keep breathing in slowly and deeply.

7. Hold onto this pose for a minute and stand with both feet on the floor.

8. After this, repeat on the other side and hold the pose for a minute.

Cobra Pose

This pose is known as bhujangasana. Lie down on your stomach and place your arms right under the shoulders. Keep your legs fully extended while your feet stay together. The top of your feet need to touch the floor. Push your chest off the floor without using your arms. If you want, you have the option to lift your hands off the ground so your body doesn't move. Your pelvis needs to always stay in contact with the floor. Hold onto this position for 2 minutes before relaxing.

Boat Pose

This is known as Navasana. Sit on your buttocks while your legs are slightly bent. Use your hands to hold the back of your knees while leaning backward. Use your bones to balance your body weight while you slowly move your arms out to the side, so they align with your knees. Ensure that your spine is elongated and straight while your chest lifts off the floor. Without changing this position, lift your toes as high as you can. Ensure that your toes are at eye level. Keep breathing in slowly and deeply while you hold onto this position for 2 minutes. Repeat this position twice.

Bridge Pose

This pose is known as Setu Bandhasana. Lie on your back while your knees are bent and placed hip-width apart. Firmly press your feet into the floor while your arms lie by your sides. As you inhale, lift your buttocks as high off the floor as you can while your pelvis stays tucked in. Your head must lie on the floor while you observe how your abdominal muscles rise and fall with every breath you inhale and exhale. Hold onto this pose for 3 minutes. As you let go, lie down on your back for 5 minutes and allow your body to relax.

Chapter 8: Ayurvedic Herbs and Aromatherapy

The therapeutic use of essential oils is known as aromatherapy. This is one of the most popular forms of holistic and natural medicines used today. It is simple to use, readily available, and pleasant. Everything in this world has a specific aroma that affects your body and mind in different ways. For instance, a lavender scent can calm your body, while the smell of cinnamon might remind you of freshly baked apple pies from childhood. Aromas are added to most cosmetics, self-care, and bath products we use. Most of us are unknowingly practicing aromatherapy. Aromatherapy is one of the therapeutic or healing techniques prescribed by Ayurveda.

Ayurvedic Aromatherapy

Aromatherapy is not a new concept and has been around for an incredibly long time. Perhaps the first form of aromatherapy known to humans was burning wood. Using aromatic smoke as a form of cleansing or burning incense is prevalent in several customs and cultures across the world. Ancient Egyptians were believed to use aromatics for over 5000 years for their medicinal and cosmetic properties, while Greeks used to mix olive oil with flower petals and herbs to absorb their fragrance and aroma. The method of distilling essential oils from plant compounds was perfected by Arab physicians, which were later introduced to Europeans.

By the 16th century, different home remedies derived from herbs aromatics gained popularity. With the increase in science and pharmacology's popularity, the widespread practice of aromatherapy faded away. It was only at the beginning of the 20th century it regained its popularity. During the beginning of the 20th century, several French chemists researched the healing properties associated with varying essential oils. The most noteworthy contributions to this field were from Rene Maurice Gattefosse. His fascination and interest in essential oils for dermatological purposes started when he discovered that lavender essential oils have healing properties. He coined the term aromatherapy in 1928, which was later published in a book under the same title.

The tradition of using dried and fresh herbs, aromatherapy oils, and floral waters is still popular in Indian and Chinese cultures. Ayurvedic physicians or vaidyas who used to treat Indian royalty often used these ingredients as therapy.

So, what are essential oils? It might seem like a buzzword or the latest trend; however, essential oils have been around for hundreds of years now. These are the highly concentrated extracts obtained from aromatic plants. Essential oils are derived from almost all parts of the plants, including flowers, bark, leaves, root, fruit, woods, and anything else imaginable. According to Ayurveda, aroma plays an important role in the prevention and healing of the human body. Aromas are used to protect prana or the life force, improve digestion and metabolism by stimulating Agni, and increase disease resistance within the body by increasing Ojas. From burning neem leaves for fumigation to bathing with water infused with rose petals, there are different ways Ayurveda incorporates essential oils and herbs. Another common practice that shows the connection between aromatherapy and Ayurveda is the burning of incense during meditation.

Use Essential Oils

Here are common practices you can follow to incorporate essential oils into your daily life.

The most straightforward way to use an essential oil is to smell it. Essential oils stimulate your sense of smell as their vapor stimulates the olfactory nerves in your body. These nerves connect your body directly to the environment and the internal workings of the brain. Several nerves and synaptic junctions the other senses involve before a specific impulse from them reaches the brain. The olfactory nerve stimulates the limbic system, and it is connected to different areas of the brain responsible for processing emotions, desires, memories, and appetite. The endocrine glands are also responsible for maintaining hormonal levels within the body and are stimulated by smells. Aromas can be subtle, but they have a significant impact on the mind and the body. This is one reason why aromatherapy is believed to be a holistic approach to treating stress. For instance, scents of rose, lavender, chamomile, sandalwood, and nutmeg can reduce the stress you experience while promoting a calming effect. These essential oils can also enhance your overall mood and promote better sleep at night.

Massage

A popular Ayurvedic technique is aromatherapy massage. You are not only inhaling these helpful aromatics, but your skin also absorbs them during a massage. The beneficial ingredients present in essential oils penetrate the skin, enter the tissues, and make their way into your body through the bloodstream. From there, they are transported to the various cells within the body. The rate of absorption is different for different oils. Regardless of all this, getting an aromatherapy massage helps stimulate, moisturize, and soothe your skin and body. A massage by itself is believed to reduce any tension present in the muscles; when you combine this with the stress-relieving properties of essential oils, the overall relaxation and calming effect increases.

Incorporate Essential Oils into Bathwater

Adding essential oils to your bath water is another critical yet straightforward way to receive oils' benefits. Soaking in a tub of warm water infused with essential oils increases your body's ability to absorb them. Warm water also reduces the stress in your muscles and promotes an overall sense of relaxation. Whether it is bath salts incorporated with essential oils or a few drops of potent essential oils, promoting overall relaxation becomes easier with this technique.

Skin and Hair Care Regime

These days, several personal care items are infused with essential oils. Essential oils are often used in shampoos, body creams and lotions, and even soaps. Depending on the overall effect you desire, choose specific essential oil. For instance, the smell of Jasmine and rose can improve your overall mood while reducing any stress you experience.

A brilliant thing about aromatherapy is it offers several applications that can be easily incorporated into your daily schedule. From diffusing essential oils to lighting an aroma candle, there is plenty to choose from. You will learn more about different essential oils ideal for balancing the three doshas in the subsequent sections.

Ayurvedic Herbs for Beginners

With aromatherapy, you need to understand Ayurvedic herbs and spices. These herbs and spices help you strengthen the connection between your body, mind, and spirit while reducing any imbalances present within. In this section, let's look at some of the best suited Ayurvedic herbs and spices for beginners.

Ashwagandha

The scientific name of ashwagandha is Withania somnifera. This is a small Woody plant native to the regions of North Africa and India. The berries and roots of this plant are commonly used in Ayurveda. Ashwagandha is believed to reduce the stress one experiences and is known to be an adaptogen. Whenever you are stressed, a hormone known as cortisol is secreted by the adrenal glands. This stress response can be reduced by using ashwagandha. It is also believed to improve your overall sleep quality, reduce stress, tackle anxiety disorders, and enhance muscle growth. Besides that, ashwagandha can improve your memory, reduce blood sugar levels, and reduce inflammation. Ashwagandha is also believed to enhance male fertility.

Boswellia

Boswellia or Indian frankincense is obtained from the resin of the Boswellia tree. It has a spicy and woody aroma believed to reduce inflammation by preventing the production of inflammatory compounds known as leukotrienes. Inflammation is beneficial in limited quantities because it is your body's first line of defense. Unfortunately, this becomes problematic when your inflammatory responses are left unregulated. Excess inflammation can cause chronic pain, reduced mobility, and an increased risk of developing rheumatoid arthritis, osteoarthritis, and other inflammatory illnesses. Inflammation can also result in breathing disorders such as asthma and digestive troubles, including ulcers. Using Boswellia can reverse this.

Triphala

Triphala is a combination of three Ayurvedic medicinal fruit, namely Indian gooseberry or Amla, bibhitaki, and haritaki. The consumption of this Ayurvedic remedy can reduce any inflammation caused by arthritis. It is also believed to act as a natural laxative that reduces abdominal pain, flatulence and improves digestion. It increases the consistency and frequency of bowel movements and reduces the risk of gut disorders. Besides this, Triphala is also used for oral care because it reduces plaque buildup, reduces the risk of gum inflammation, and the presence of undesirable bacteria in the mouth.

Brahmi

The scientific name of Brahmi is bacopa monieri, and it is commonly used in Ayurvedic remedies. The anti-inflammatory properties of this herb can combat inflammation present in the body. Instead of depending on pharmaceuticals with various side effects, it's always better to opt for Ayurvedic remedies derived from natural sources. If you want to improve your attention span, memory, and learning rate, using Brahmi is a good idea. It is also believed to promote self-control, reduce restlessness, and increase impulse regulation. The adaptogen properties of Brahmi enhance your body's ability to deal with mental and physical stress.

Cumin

Cumin is a spice often used in Asian and Mediterranean cooking. It is native to the regions of South West Asia and the Mediterranean. The seeds from the cumin plant have a spicy and nutty aroma and flavor. It is used as a home remedy to improve the digestive process. Cumin increases the activity of digestive enzymes that facilitate the sufficient production of bile from the liver. In turn, this speeds up the process of digestion while enhancing your body's ability to digest fats in the food consumed. It can reduce the symptoms of irritable bowel syndrome, including bloating and pain. It is believed to improve insulin sensitivity while reducing the levels of blood sugar. When you put both these factors together, it becomes an effective remedy to reduce Type 2 diabetes risk factors. The antimicrobial properties of humans reduce the risk of foodborne illness.

Turmeric

Turmeric or Golden spice is an incredibly popular Ayurvedic remedy. The active compound in turmeric is known as curcumin. The anti-inflammatory and antioxidant properties associated with turmeric are due to the presence of curcumin. It's believed to enhance blood flow, improve the function of brain-derived neurotrophic factor, and reduce inflammation. When you put these factors together, turmeric can reduce the risk of heart disease and neurodegenerative disorders.

Licorice Root

Licorice root is obtained from the Glycyrrhiza glabra plant and is native to the regions of Asia and Europe and is often used in Ayurvedic remedies. Licorice root is believed to strengthen your immune response and help fight various pathogens, including bacteria and viruses. Apart from that, licorice also reduces inflammation within your body. It is used to relieve the symptoms of a sore throat while improving oral health. Besides that, it's used in Ayurveda to reduce certain digestive troubles such as bloating, ulcers, belching, and nausea. It can also be used topically to reduce skin irritation such as redness, swelling, rash, and itching.

Bitter Melon

The scientific name of bitter melon is Momordica charantia. It's a tropical vegetable native to the Asian region and is quite similar to vegetables that grow on vines such as pumpkins and squash. It is filled with helpful nutrients and anti-inflammatory compounds. Bitter melon can reduce your blood sugar levels while promoting the secretion and functioning of insulin. Insulin is the hormone responsible for stabilizing your blood sugar levels. It's also believed to reduce the levels of harmful cholesterol.

Cardamom is known as the Queen of spices, and its scientific name is Elettaria cardamommum. It's been a part of Ayurvedic remedies since time immemorial. Besides reducing blood pressure, cardamom essential oil can increase your body's ability to utilize oxygen during exercise. Cardamom can also reduce digestive trouble such as gastric ulcers and offer better protection to the gut bacteria.

Aromatherapy for Tridoshas

Depending on your Prakriti, the type of essential oils you use will also differ. Those with Vata Prakriti or vikruti benefit from warming oils that have a calming effect. Such oils usually have a sweet or pungent rasa, sweet vipaka, and warm virya. The most common blends of sweet and spicy aromatics help to pacify the Vata dosha. The sweet scent brings a sense of calm while the spicy aroma warms up your body from the inside. For instance, sandalwood and cinnamon can be mixed to create a spicy-sweet blend for Vata dosha.

Similarly, cooling oils are ideal for those with pita vikruti or Prakriti. The aromas of essential oils used to rebalance Pitta dosha usually have a sweet rasa, sweet vipaka, and cool virya. Those with Kapha vikruti or Prakriti benefit from oils slightly warm and simulating. Most of the essential oils used for balancing Kapha dosha are spicy or pungent. There pungent rasa, pungent vipaka, and warm virya help stimulate and clear the mind.

The essential oils and aromas ideal for Vata dosha include basil, lavender, camphor, rose, and sandalwood. Honeysuckle, lavender, rose, and sandalwood are ideal for Pitta dosha. The Kapha dosha benefits from camphor, basil, Wintergreen, patchouli, cedar, and sage essential oils and aromas.

Chapter 9: Panchakarma: The Ayurvedic Detox

Ayurveda's primary focus is on preventative and healing therapies or techniques that promote purification and rejuvenation of your body, mind, and spirit. It is more than a holistic healing system. It is all about following healthy lifestyle patterns and a diet that restores balance in your body, consciousness, and mind. This preventive and healing technique reduces the risk of any illnesses or diseases.

The five basic elements of the universe manifest themselves in the form of three doshas that are present in all our bodies. Everyone has a unique elemental composition determined by the three doshas' proportions at the time of birth or fertilization. An individual's constitution is determined as soon as the embryo is formed in the mother's womb. Each of us has all three doshas in varying proportions. According to Ayurveda, by using different permutations and combinations, there are seven primary constitutions of doshas in humans. These constitutions are as follows.

- Predominant Vata
- Predominant pitta
- Predominant Kapha

- Predominant Vata-pitta
- Predominant pitta- Kapha
- Predominant pitta-Vata
- Equal balance in Vata, pitta, and Kapha

By now, you have probably understood that every individual has a specific and unique composition of Vata, pitta, and Kapha dosha. Balancing these three doshas is the natural order of the universe. If this balance between doshas is disturbed, it creates a sense of disorder and imbalance. If health is associated with the order, the disease is equivalent to disorder. There exists a constant interaction between order and disorder within your body. You can reestablish order by understanding the structure and the nature of the disorder present within. According to Ayurveda, there is always order even within a disorder. All that required is conscious attention.

According to Ayurveda, the order is defined as the state of health. When your digestive fire or Agni is well balanced, there exists order. Similarly, when your physiological energies of Vata, pitta, and Kapha are in equilibrium, there is order. The three waste products produced by the body- urine, sweat, and feces - are produced and eliminated properly, then there is order within. There are seven bodily tissues: rasa, rakta, mamsa, asthi, meda, majja, and artava. If all these are functioning normally, it is a sign of order. The order can also be described as a state when your body, mind, senses, and spirit or consciousness work synergistically and in harmony. An imbalance in relationships results in disorder.

Vata, Pitta, and Kapha doshas regulate the internal environment of your body. These energies are constantly interacting with the external environment and are creating internal reactions. Different factors can cause imbalances in all these tridoshas. From following the wrong diet to unhealthy lifestyle habits and consuming incompatible food combinations, these doshas' function is affected. Besides this, improper stress management, suppressing and repressing your emotions, and not dealing with seasonal changes properly can also result in an imbalance of three doshas. For instance, it was previously mentioned that every meal you consume needs to be a combination of six tastes. However, certain foods don't pair well together. Certain foods, such as milk and fish, yogurt, and meat, should not be paired together. Cooked honey should not be consumed. Depending on the nature of the cause of imbalance, the three doshas are aggravated or disarranged. The effect of both these things is the same. It ultimately results in negatively affecting the digestive fire or Agni. When Agni can't function like it is supposed to, it increases the production of ama or toxins.

When there is an excess buildup of ama in the body, they enter the bloodstream. Once they enter the bloodstream, these toxins are circulated to all the cells. This prevents proper cellular function and clogs various channels within the body. Toxemia occurs when there is the retention of toxins in the blood. When your body is functioning properly, it keeps expelling toxins from within while preventing recovery. If all these toxins are not regularly removed and they accumulate, it slowly but affects your vital life energy known as prana. It also reduces cellular energy while reducing Ojas or immunity. When you put all this together, it increases your body's susceptibility to disease while preventing its overall function. Every disease is often a crisis of excess toxicity in the body. The internal cause of all diseases is ama. The aggravated dosha always causes ama. Understanding all this brings you a step closer to increasing your body's ability to prevent disease.

The simplest thing you can do is enable your body's natural ability to eliminate toxins to prevent disease. To prevent further production of ama while increasing its elimination, it follows that a proper diet while making appropriate lifestyle changes works. Besides consuming a dosha balancing diet, make healthy habits such as regular exercise and a proper sleep schedule a part of your daily routine. Now, your work doesn't just end there. Follow a regular detoxifying program to enhance your body's overall function. This cleansing or detoxifying process is known as panchakarma. Panchakarma is a combination of two Sanskrit words, Pancha and karma. Pancha means five, while karma means treatments or actions. Panchakarma means a 5-step process that involves detoxification of your body from the inside. Your body needs to be detoxified, so it does not suffer from the adverse effects of poor lifestyle choices and environmental pollution.

Panchakarma helps restore your body's natural healing capacity while improving your overall health. When your body can heal itself, its function improves naturally. By complementing the process of panchakarma with meditation and yoga, you can reestablish and strengthen the natural connection between your body, mind, and spirit. When these three aspects of your life are in harmony with one another, your overall sense of wellbeing will improve.

Who wouldn't want to lead a healthier life? Unfortunately, the modern concept of leading a healthy life is riddled with pharmaceuticals and synthetic cures that only treat the symptoms of any disease or disorder we experience. If all you do is treat the symptom, the actual cause of it is left untreated. This, in turn, increases the chances of the disease or disorder reappearing. This is where Ayurveda steps into the picture. Instead of merely treating the symptoms, Ayurveda delves deeper and tries to tackle the disease's cause. When the disease is addressed at its grassroots level, its recurrence will be minimized. Ayurveda is also focused on preventive care instead of just curative care, which is often full of chemical concoctions. Instead of following a crash diet or using the health fads that keep coming up, it's better to go back to the basics. Natural remedies and preventive techniques are always better than chemical and pharmaceutical cures. After all, prevention is better than the cure.

Panchakarma treatments are created to work along with your body's natural ability to process and remove the presence of toxins from the inside. It helps purify and heal your body from the inside without wearing itself down. Your body can't function optimally if you consume a poor diet, lead a stressful life, and use unhealthy coping mechanisms such as the consumption of alcohol or drugs to deal with stress.

A panchakarma treatment lays down the primary foundation for a cleaner body, which is a sign of good health. It restores your body to its original state of functioning, where it is free from all toxins. By undergoing this process, you are eliminating toxins and imbalances present within. When your body is restored to its original form, overall health and vitality increase. You can't build a house on a foundation infested with termites. The only way to build a strong and sturdy house is by laying down a solid foundation. This is how Ayurveda works. Ayurvedic panchakarma helps rebuild, restore, and rejuvenate your body.

While following the Ayurvedic practices, you will realize that they're often preventive. It helps stop most illnesses from manifesting by helping you lead a healthy life. Panchakarma is a periodic detoxification and cleansing process, which ensures your system is working and stays in good order. It prevents the accumulation of disease-causing toxins while strengthening internal mechanisms. Ayurvedic teachings detect imbalances and then eliminate them. Unfortunately, most of us are already afflicted with varying disorders and even serious chronic ailments. By choosing Ayurvedic panchakarma treatment, you can cope with several severe diseases.

Common medical cases can be treated with panchakarma. Problems with blood circulation and hypertension or cardiac disorders benefit from a panchakarma treatment. It's used to alleviate respiratory problems, including asthma, allergies, and colds, gastrointestinal problems, joint disease, dermatological illnesses, and fertility problems. Panchakarma helps rebalance your body and bring it back to its original state of function, which is a great way to eliminate psychological imbalances and even insomnia. All in all, panchakarma helps increase your sense of wellbeing and health.

Your body has an inbuilt detoxifying system. When it is overworked or not working as intended, it increases your susceptibility to disease and illness. Ayurveda and panchakarma therapies restore your body's natural healing ability while improving your immunity. All this is done by cleansing and restoring the natural detoxification system. As with any other non-surgical cure, it will take time to see the benefits associated with panchakarma, but you will notice a significant change in your overall health over a period. Before you undergo a panchakarma treatment, you need to find a good Ayurvedic practitioner certified to assess you and help by prescribing treatment according to your needs and requirements.

Panchakarma is divided into two steps. The first step is known as poova karma, and the second step is known as pradhan karma. Pradhan karma is further divided into five steps. During poova karma, the patient is prepared mentally and physically for the panchakarma processes. Poova karma includes simply processing, which helps the liquefaction of fat-soluble toxins in the body. It essentially consists of three processes designed to enhance the overall detoxification effects of panchakarma.

Poova karma includes pachan karma, snehan karma, and swedan karma. Pachan karma includes fasting and consuming Ayurvedic herbs that liquefy the fat-soluble toxins present within the cells. During snehan karma, you will be administered gradually increasing doses of Ayurvedic or medicated ghee to stimulate the liquefaction of fat-soluble toxins deep within the tissues. The final stage of poova karma is a deep tissue Ayurvedic massage and steam bath that opens the pores to eliminate toxins.

Once you undergo poova karma, it brings us to the next stage, which includes five steps to facilitate total detoxification. The five steps in the Pradhan karma are vamanam, virechanam, basti, nasya, and raktamokshana. Vamanam includes induced vomiting, which helps clear the toxins present in the upper part of the gastrointestinal tract and the respiratory tract. Virechanam refers to purgation, which helps clear the lower gastrointestinal tract - the region from the stomach to the excretory system. Basti refers to an herbal oil enema that helps clear lipid waste from the rectal region while nasya or nasal irrigation clears the respiratory tract and sinuses. The final stage is raktamokshana, where a certified Ayurvedic practitioner lets out impure blood.

If your Ayurvedic composition is dominated by Vata dosha, add a pinch of rock salt to ghee, while Kapha will benefit from adding a pinch of trikatu. Don't forget to follow a dosha balancing diet. Before you go to sleep at night, add one teaspoon of Triphala powder to ½ cup of water and let it boil. Drink this concoction ten minutes before you go to bed. This acts as a mild laxative that helps detoxify your digestive system. You need to follow this routine for the first three days of the panchakarma.

Tips for Panchakarma at Home

The good news is you don't necessarily have to go to an Ayurvedic retreat to follow a panchakarma routine. Instead, there are simple practices you can use to perform panchakarma at home. In the section, you can learn about it.

Before you get started with panchakarma, it's important to understand your Ayurvedic constitution. Your Ayurvedic constitution is determined by the presence of three doshas in your body. Most of us have a primary dosha and other secondary and less prominent doshas. Unless you understand this, you can't create a panchakarma routine that is good for you. All the information you need to determine your Ayurvedic constitution was described in detail in the previous chapters.

Before you start a panchakarma routine, it is important to take a break from your usual lifestyle. Spend time to get all the rest your body needs, walk in nature, and practice yoga and meditation. Think of it as a weeklong vacation where you escape the stress of your daily grind. Avoid activities that result in excess stimulation, spend time outdoors, and get all the rest you need. While practicing panchakarma, there is one important step you need to remember. It can cause the release of old, repressed, and unresolved emotions stored within your subconscious. Whenever you are detoxifying your body, be prepared to detoxify your mind and emotions too. After taking a break from your daily lifestyle, it is time to get started with panchakarma.

While following the panchakarma routine at home, it can be extended over 12 days. Here is a sample of what these 12 days will look like.

Days 1-3

Start the day by drinking two ounces of warm ghee when you wake up in the morning. Wake up at sunrise and sleep at sunset. If your blood sugar or blood pressure is high, replace ghee with two tablespoons of flaxseed. Consume two-tablespoon flaxseed 15 minutes before every meal for three days.

If your Ayurvedic composition is dominated by Vata dosha, add a pinch of rock salt to ghee, while Kapha will benefit from adding a pinch of trikatu. Don't forget to follow a dosha balancing diet. Before you sleep at night, add one teaspoon of Triphala powder to ½ cup of water and let it boil. Drink this concoction ten minutes before you go to bed. This acts as a mild laxative that helps detoxify your digestive system. You need to follow this routine for the first three days of the panchakarma.

Days 4-5

Consume a khichdi or kitchhari for breakfast, lunch, and dinner during these three days. Khichdi or kitchhari is a mild dish made of softly cooked lentils and rice. Drink dosha-specific freshly brewed teas on these days. Here are the Ayurvedic powders you can make for each of the three doshas.

Vata dosha - mix ground cumin, ginger, and coriander in equal portions. Mix equal portions of ground cumin, fennel, and coriander for Pitta dosha and equal parts of ground ginger cinnamon for Kapha dosha.

15-20 minutes before bedtime, massage your body with organic oil. For Vata dosha, use sesame oil while sunflower and corn oils are good for Pitta and Kapha doshas, respectively. Let your skin absorb this oil for a couple of minutes, and then take a hot bath before sleeping. Don't forget to drink the Triphala concoction described in the previous step.

Days 6-8

Stick to the daily diet of khichdi and tea followed by evening massage, shower, and Triphala during these two days. There is one addition you need to make now. Right before you go to bed, add 1 tsp of dashamoola to 2 cups of water and let it boil for five minutes. Once this brew has cooled down, strain it and use the liquid as a basti. Ideally, you should retain this brew liquid for 30 minutes before heading to the bathroom.

Days 9-12

The main panchakarma has come to an end. On the ninth day, you can add steamed vegetables to your daily meal of khichdi. Gradually add more vegetables and unyeasted bread to your diet. Don't stop following a dosha-specific Ayurvedic diet after the panchakarma if you want to maintain the benefits obtained so far.

Chapter 10: Incorporating Ayurveda Into Your Life

You have now been introduced to different concepts of Ayurveda and the benefits they offer. Now that you are armed with all the information you need, it's time to incorporate Ayurveda into your daily lifestyle. By now, you will have realized that it is so much more than a holistic system of healing. Instead, it is the key to leading a healthier and happier life by balancing different elements of your physiological composition.

Helpful Ayurvedic Lifestyle Tips

To obtain the various benefits of Ayurveda discussed in the previous chapters, here are simple tips you can follow.

Following an Ayurvedic Diet

In the previous sections, you were introduced to the philosophies and basic principles of an Ayurvedic diet. The Ayurvedic diet is an effective way to improve your overall health and wellbeing. It can be easily customized according to your physiological constitution of doshas. Depending on the predominant doshas, you can choose foods that increase Ojas while reducing ama. In turn, it rebalances your energy while ensuring that your body gets all the nutrients it needs. An Ayurvedic diet is predominantly plant-based and is rich and all the macro and micronutrients your body needs for its effective functioning. Once you become mindful of the foods you consume, making healthier choices becomes more effortless.

Home-Cooked Meals

Try to avoid eating out as much as you can. Avoid ready-to-cook meals and instead cook your meals at home. This is not only a great way of ensuring that your body gets all the essential nutrients it needs, but it strengthens your connection with the food you eat. When you know where the ingredients come from and put effort into cooking your meal, you are more mindful of your diet and appetite. Home-cooked meals are not only more nutritious and healthier, but they are also light on your pocket in the long run. This is something your bank balance will thank you for!

Avoid Processed Foods

A prominent characteristic of Ayurvedic eating is that it limits your consumption of processed and packaged foods. These are unhealthy, devoid of nutrients, and are a leading cause of weight gain. Even if you feel like snacking, choose healthier alternatives instead of a packet of crisps or cookies. Aside from processed and packaged food, become mindful of your consumption of processed sugars and artificial sweeteners. Sugar is extremely inflammatory and aggravates or triggers metabolic disorders. Shift to natural sources of sugar such as fruit and fruit juices instead of munching on unhealthy snacks.

Stay Hydrated

It is not only important to pay attention to the food you consume, but hydration matters too. You need to drink around 7-8 glasses of water daily. Drink more if required. Water cleanses your body from the inside while promoting better function of the digestive system. Drinking sufficient water will improve your overall energy levels while hydrating your skin and hair. If you are not used to drinking water regularly, set the alarm, or use an online application to do this.

Increase Your Intake of Herbal Teas

If you can't do away with your morning cup of coffee and need a warm beverage to wake yourself up, choose herbal teas. Instead of coffee, replace it with herbal tea sweetened using natural sweeteners. You can consume herbal teas between your meals instead of munching on unnecessary snacks. It acts as an appetite stimulant while improving the function of your digestive system.

Make Time for a Detox

The Ayurvedic practice of panchakarma was explained in detail in the previous chapter. Detoxifying your body helps enhance its overall function while optimizing your health and sense of wellbeing. Detoxification is important to strengthen your physical and mental function. By making time for a detox, you are essentially improving your health.

Oil Your Hair

Don't forget to oil your hair at least once a week. Massaging your scalp with warm oil stimulates your nerves while promoting blood supply to the hair. If you like the idea of a healthier, shiny, and full mane, oiling your hair at least once a week is essential. Always massage your scalp with warm oil instead of normal room temperature oil.

Engage in Physical Activity

You need to make a conscious effort to add physical activity to your daily routine. Whether it is going to the gym or running, physical activity is crucial for your overall health and wellbeing. Regular physical activity improves your mental, physical, and emotional health. The best way to do this is by practicing yoga daily. Using the different yoga poses discussed in the previous chapters, you can harmonize the tridosha on your body. So, it is not just your physical health that improves. Your elemental composition also functions like it's supposed to.

Declutter Your Space

Decluttering your physical surroundings is as important as decluttering your mind. Meditation helps declutter your mind and make space for positivity. Similarly, by decluttering your surroundings, you can make space for desirable things needed in your life. Take stock of your surroundings, note all the objects and items that add value to your life while noticing if there are things you don't need or that add no value to your life. Get rid of them immediately. Unless you eliminate clutter, you can't accommodate desirable things.

Spend Time Outdoors

Spend time outdoors. Reconnecting with nature is a great way to improve your overall sense of wellbeing. Most of us live in a concrete jungle or are leading such hectic lives we don't appreciate nature's beauty. Take time and reconnect with nature daily. It can be something as simple as going to your local park or meditating while sitting under a tree. Walking barefoot on the grass can be quite a good stress buster.

Make the Most of the Time Available

Forget about any mistakes or regrets of the past and worry about the future. Neither thing is in your control. The only thing you have is this moment so learn to make the most of the time available. Become grateful for the present and concentrate on creating a future you desire. Practicing gratitude helps leverage the power of the law of attraction. When you are thankful for all the good you have in life, it sends a message to the universe there is room for good in your life. Maintain a positive attitude, monitor your internal self-talk, and adopt a positive attitude toward life and yourself. When you feel good about yourself, it shows in your thoughts, actions, and behaviors.

Practice Breathing Exercises

Practice daily breathing exercises. Breathing exercises are meditative and help calm your mind. The great thing about this is you can do it wherever and whenever you want. Whenever you feel stressed or overwhelmed, take a break from the activity you are engaged in, find a quiet spot, and concentrate on breathing. This helps calm your mind and regulate your thoughts.

Eliminate Negativity from Your Life

Remember, you have complete control over the kind of energy you let into your life. Become mindful of any toxic or harmful energy in your surroundings. If interacting with someone drains your energy or makes you feel negative, it's a sign of a toxic relationship. Eliminate all negativity sources from your life, and if elimination isn't possible, distance yourself from toxic individuals. The simplest way to do this is by becoming mindful of your feelings and emotions around different people and places. If something doesn't feel good or it feels off, you probably are right.

Sleep Cycle

Learn to regularize your sleep schedule. Wake up early, sleep early, and stick to this routine. It might not come easily to you, but it is good for your overall health and wellbeing in the long run. By resynchronizing your sleep cycle with the sunset and sunrise, you are strengthening your natural biological clock's functioning, known as the circadian rhythm.

Morning and Evening Routine

Apart from all the tips shown above, you need to establish a morning and evening routine to ensure that you make the most of the 24-hours available. This allows you to plan your days and make time for yourself. Planning is important for time management. You will learn about this in the next sections.

A Morning Routine

Time is a limited resource; learning to make the most of it is vital to achieving your life goals. The simplest way to do this is by creating a healthy daily routine that reestablishes the connection between your body, mind, and spirit. Ayurveda places importance on the need for a proper morning routine. By establishing an ideal routine, you can regularize your circadian rhythm, improve digestion, and promote the absorption of nutrients while optimizing assimilation. Apart from this, a productive morning routine increases your self-discipline, happiness, and even self-esteem. In this section, let's look at an ideal morning routine that incorporates the teachings of Ayurveda.

Wake Up Early

Early to bed and early to rise makes a man healthy, wealthy, and wise. This saying is true, and the sooner you start living by it, the better it is for overall health and wellbeing. Ideally, our bodies are synchronized with the sunrise and sunset patterns. Waking up before sunrise helps refresh your senses while increasing your peace of mind. Even though the sunrise timings vary depending on your location, the ideal time to wake up is around 6:00 AM. As soon as you wake up, take a couple of moments, and look at your hands. Gently move them over your face, neck, chest, and waist. It is a simple way to cleanse your aura in the morning.

A Little Spirituality Helps

Whether you are religious or not, getting in touch with your spirituality always helps. Spirituality and religion are not synonymous. You can be spiritual without believing in a specific religion. If you want, pray to a deity before leaving your bed. Alternatively, you can seek the guidance of the cosmos to help you get through the day and make the most of the opportunities that come your way. Energy is abundant in the cosmos, and unless you seek its guidance, it will not help you.

Clean Your Face

After you have sent out a small prayer, it's time to splash cold water on your face. Don't forget to wash your mouth and eyes with it. Gently massage your eyelids and blink your eyes seven times while rotating them in different directions. Wipe your face with a soft and dry cloth.

Drink a cup of water after you've cleaned your face, mouth, and eyes. Drink a glass of water at room temperature. Ayurveda suggests that drinking from a cup made of pure copper helps. Fill this cup with water before you go to sleep and drink it at room temperature after cleansing your face in the morning. It helps cleanse your gastrointestinal tract and flush toxins from the kidneys. Even if you are used to starting a new day with a cup of tea or coffee, avoid it. This habit usually increases the stress on your kidneys and adrenaline glands, which prevents your body's digestive system from functioning effectively.

Time for Evacuation

The ideal position for having a bowel movement is by sitting or squatting on the toilet seat. You can regulate your bowel movements by having a glass of water in the morning and using the washroom at the same time every day. You can also practice alternate nostril breathing to improve the body's ability to evacuate the previous night's meal. Don't forget to wash the anal orifice with warm water after evacuation. The last step is to wash your hands thoroughly with soap.

A Healthy Oral Routine

Scraping your tongue in a back-forth motion helps cover its entire surface. You need to do this 7-14 times to cleanse your tongue thoroughly. Scraping your tongue stimulates your digestive system, internal organs, promotes suggestion and removes harmful bacteria from your mouth cavity. A stainless-steel scraper is the best one available for all doshas. If you are more dosha specific, use a gold scraper for Vata dosha, a silver one for Pitta, and copper for Kapha.

Once you have scraped your tongue, it's time to brush your teeth. Always use a soft-bristle toothbrush and a pungent, bitter, or astringent toothpaste or tooth powder. Traditionally, neem twigs were used as toothbrushes in ancient India. The antibacterial properties of neem strengthen the gums and remove any food particles or bacteria present in the mouth.

Now, it is time to gargle. Gargling strengthens your voice, teeth, gums, and jaw. Gargle at least twice a day. Using warm sesame oil to gargle is an ancient Ayurvedic remedy. Hold this oil in your mouth, switch it around vigorously twice, and spit it out. Gently massage your gums to strengthen them. This brings us to the end of the oral routine.

Chew Mindfully

Strengthen and improve your teeth and gum health by chewing on a handful of raw sesame seeds. You can also chew an inch of dried coconut or three dried dates. This stimulates your digestive system and stokes Agni or digestive fire. After chewing, brush your teeth once again.

Exercise Routine

The ideal time to exercise is early in the morning when your body and mind are fresh. Engaging in any form of physical activity is good for your wellbeing. To enhance its benefits further, practice yoga regularly. Follow the different suggestions about yoga position-specific for doshas was mentioned in the previous chapter. Use that information to improve your blood circulation, stamina, strength, and vitality. Regular exercise also increases your overall sense of relaxation and promotes a good quality of sleep at night.

Apart from exercise, take time for meditation and breathing exercises. Meditating for as little as 10-15 minutes daily, especially during the morning hours, promotes mental clarity. Now is the time to align your thoughts and create a to-do list for the day that lies ahead. Instead of going about your day like a headless chicken, meditating early in the morning helps you concentrate on your goals and ensures better time management when you know what needs to be done and when your ability to get things done improves.

Use Nasal Drops

Using nasal drops helps lubricate the nasal passage, clear the sinuses, increase mental clarity, and enhance your vision and voice. The olfactory senses have a direct connection to the brain. So, taking care of it helps improve your mental function. Warm ghee or oil can be used as nasal drops. You need about 3-5 drops of this to cleanse your nasal passage. Ghee is ideal for all doshas, while sesame oil, coconut oil, and calamus root oil are ideal for Vata, pitta, and Kapha doshas, respectively.

Concentrate on the Ears

Excess Vata in the ears can present itself as excess earwax, difficulty in hearing, lockjaw, or even a constant ringing in the ears. To prevent this, put a few drops of warm sesame oil in the ears.

Massage Your Head and Body with Oil

Make it a point to massage your head and body using warm oil. Massage your scalp with oil to prevent headaches, graying of hair, and reduce the chances of a receding hairline. Before you go to sleep, massage your body with a little warm oil to promote sleep quality. Oil massage also keeps your skin feeling soft, supple and gives it a youthful look. Use sunflower or coconut oil for Pitta dosha, sesame oil for Vata dosha, and master sunflower oil for Kapha dosha.

Bath Time

Taking a bath daily is not only cleansing and refreshing, but it leaves you feeling energetic. Bathing with warm water or water infused with essential oils ideal for your dosha promotes cleanliness while bringing mental clarity. While bathing, take your time cleaning every part of your body, and don't rush.

Take Pride in Your Attire

To promote your overall sense of wellbeing and self-confidence, always wear clean clothes. To practice better time management, choose your outfit the previous night so you don't waste time in the morning. Using perfumes and body care products infused with essential oils can improve your overall sense of wellbeing. The information in the previous chapter about aromatherapy and Ayurveda will help you find the right essential oil for your dosha.

Once you have followed all the steps, it's time for breakfast. Never keep your stomach empty, especially after exercise in the morning. All these stored energies from the previous night will have been extinguished by now. Have a light breakfast and get a head start on your day.

By following this healthy morning routine, you can improve your overall sense of wellbeing. It also helps strengthen the bond between your body, mind, and soul.

Evening Routine

How you end each day is as important as how you start it. Most of us are too focused on creating an ideal morning routine that we forget about an evening routine. If you struggle to unwind, especially after a long and tiring day, establish a healthy evening routine. Whether it's morning or evening, routines ensure optimal utilization of time. Most of us believe that watching TV or spending time in front of an electronic gadget is a great way to relax. Instead, this merely increases the stress on your internal systems. An ideal way to relax is by taking time for yourself. According to Ayurvedic teachings, a healthy evening routine helps rebalance your life and bring about a sense of stability and peace. It can be a little tricky to create and maintain a new routine but do not get overwhelmed. With a little conscious effort, you can create and maintain a healthy evening routine.

Yoga and Meditation

You might be wondering why you need to engage in more yoga if you have already practiced it in the morning. The importance of yoga can never be overlooked when it comes to your health and wellbeing. Regardless of how tiring your day gets, engaging in a little yoga is good for you. You don't need an elaborate yoga or meditation routine. Instead, concentrate on the yoga and meditation suggestions in the previous chapters, which were ideal for dosha balancing. Engaging in this practice for as little as 15- 20 minutes in the evening can calm your body, mind, and spirit.

Pay Attention to Your Meal

According to Ayurvedic teachings, you need to consume the heaviest meal of the day at noon. Your body's internal fire or Agni starts slowing down as you near bedtime, so consume light and easy to digest food. Your dinnertime should be such that you give your body a break for at least three hours before you go to sleep. This ensures optimal digestion and better absorption of nutrients. Avoid any heavy foods and, instead, opt for a light dinner. Ideally, choose plant-based foods instead of animal-based ones if you want to rebalance your doshas and ensure your body gets the nourishment it needs.

Time for Leisure

Most of us lead hectic lives these days, and we need to schedule a time for winding down too. It might sound counterintuitive that you need to plan to take a break. Unless you plan, chances are you will keep ignoring it. After dinner:

1. Spend time enjoying an activity or hobby you love.

2. Do not use this time to sit in front of a bright screen.

3. Take a break from all blue light-emitting devices.

Blue light stimulates your mind, increases stress, and prevents melatonin, a sleep-inducing hormone, from working its magic. To sleep at night, avoid screen time after dinner. Instead, go for a walk, listen to soothing music, and spend as little time on the artificial light as possible.

Have a Warm Drink

Before you go to bed, make it a practice to have a warm drink. Consuming a warm beverage, especially warm milk, improves your ability to fall asleep at night. It also encourages your mind to disengage from any stress it experiences. Consuming a cup of warm milk infused with turmeric or saffron can work wonders for your sleep cycle. If you want to add honey to this, ensure that you do it after the milk has cooled down. Heating or cooking honey removes its beneficial properties while making it difficult for your body to digest.

Massaging your body and head with warm oil before going to sleep promotes overall relaxation while thoroughly moisturizing your head and body. The calming effect of rubbing warm oil on your body goes a long way to improving your sleep quality at night.

Bedtime

You must sleep and wake up at the same time every day. Ensure that you don't stay up late and do the night and go to sleep before 10:00 pm; if you sleep early, your ability to wake up earlier in the morning increases. Sleeping late and waking up early will harm your overall health eventually. Go to bed at the same time every day, whether or not it's a weekday or a holiday. Consistency is important for developing and maintaining a habit.

By following all these simple suggestions, you can easily create an evening routine designed to improve your overall sense of wellbeing. When you take care of your body, mind, and soul, your overall health will automatically improve. Ayurveda is all about creating sustainable habits.

All the suggestions discussed in this chapter are easy to follow. However, don't try to do everything at once. Instead, gradually incorporate these steps into your daily routine and strive to create healthier yet sustainable habits. Ayurveda is not a short-term solution. It is the key to a better lifestyle. Be patient and do not rush into it. Trust this process and work toward inculcating healthier lifestyle habits. Now, all that's left for you to do is get started immediately. If you are patient, consistent, and conscious and all the effort you make, you will notice a positive change within no time.

Conclusion

Ayurveda is the ancient science of healing. From improving your energy levels to reducing the risk of illnesses and managing any pre-existing health conditions, the holistic approach of Ayurveda is well rounded. It is the key to improving your overall health. This is one of the leading reasons people worldwide are turning to this natural therapy to improve their health.

The philosophy of Ayurveda includes a variety of systems specifically designed to deal with different health conditions and aspects of your health. This holistic approach helps rebalance your body, mind, soul, and senses. By using Ayurveda, you can improve the overall quality of your life. In this book, you were given everything you need to incorporate the simple practice of Ayurveda into your lifestyle. From becoming mindful of your diet to yoga and meditation, you can balance and heal your internal systems. Once your body starts functioning effectively and optimally, your health will improve. Whether it is your mental or physical wellbeing, Ayurveda has all the answers you need.

Now, all that's left for you to do is start following the simple and practical tips and suggestions in this book. The key to your overall wellbeing lies in your hands. The sooner you start, the better.

Here's another book by Mari Silva that you might like

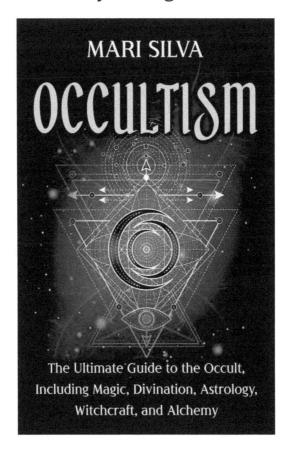

Your Free Gift (only available for a limited time)

Thanks for getting this book! If you want to learn more about various spirituality topics, then join Mari Silva's community and get a free guided meditation MP3 for awakening your third eye. This guided meditation mp3 is designed to open and strengthen ones third eye so you can experience a higher state of consciousness. Simply visit the link below the image to get started.

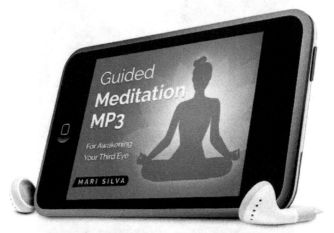

https://spiritualityspot.com/meditation

References

25 Actionable Ayurvedic Lifestyle Tips to Live Ayurveda Life. (2019, November 2). Retreat Kula website: Https://retreatkula.com/blog/ayurvedic-lifestyle-tips/

Ali, S. (2020, December 6). The Two Supplements An Herbalist Wants You To Take To Stop Fall Allergies in Their Tracks. Well+Good website: Https://www.wellandgood.com/supplements-fight-allergies/

Ayurveda - Basic Principles. (n.d.). Ayurherbs Clinic Melbourne website: Https://www.ayurherbs.com.au/principles-of-ayurveda/

Ayurvedic Medicine: History and Principles. (n.d.). Copper H2O website:

https://www.copperh2o.com/blogs/blog/ayurvedic-medicine-origin-history-and-principles

Basso, J. C., McHale, A., Ende, V., Oberlin, D. J., & Suzuki, W. A. (2019). Brief, daily meditation enhances attention, memory, mood, and emotional regulation in non-experienced meditators. Behavioral brain research, 356, 208–220. https://www.sciencedirect.com/science/article/abs/pii/S016643281830322X?via%3Dihub

Easterly, E. (2019, September 10). 10 Rules for an Ayurvedic Diet. Chopra website: Https://chopra.com/articles/10-rules-for-an-ayurvedic-diet

Easterly, E. (2020, March 3). Ayurveda Doshas: The Benefit of Knowing Your Unique Dosha. Chopra website: Https://chopra.com/articles/ayurveda-doshas-the-benefit-of-knowing-your-unique-dosha

Elements in Ayurveda and their Significance | YO1 Health Resort, Catskills. (n.d.). www.yo1.com website: Https://www.yo1.com/health-guide/elements-in-ayurveda-and-their-significance.html

Fiolet, T., Srour, B., Sellem, L., Kesse-Guyot, E., Allès, B., Méjean, C., Deschasaux, M., Fassier, P., Latino-Martel, P., Beslay, M., Hercberg, S., Lavalette, C., Monteiro, C. A., Julia, C., & Touvier, M. (2018). Consumption of ultra-processed foods and cancer risk: results from NutriNet-Santé prospective cohort. BMJ (Clinical research ed.), 360, k322. https://www.bmj.com/content/360/bmj.k322

Galante, J., Galante, I., Bekkers, M. J., & Gallacher, J. (2014). Effect of kindness-based meditation on health and wellbeing: a systematic review and meta-analysis. Journal of consulting and clinical psychology, 82(6), 1101–1114. https://doi.apa.org/doiLanding?doi=10.1037%2Fa0037249

Gerson, S. (2019, January 13). Ayurveda and the Chakras by Scott Gerson, M.D., M.Phil. (Ayurveda), Ph.D. (Ayurveda). GIAM website: https://www.gersonayurveda.com/giam-blog/2019/1/6/ayurveda-and-the-chakras-by-scott-gerson-md-mphil-ayurveda-phd-ayurveda

Giovanni. (2015, April 14). What is Meditation? Live and Dare website: https://liveanddare.com/what-is-meditation/

Goyal, M., Singh, S., Sibinga, E. M., Gould, N. F., Rowland-Seymour, A., Sharma, R., Berger, Z., Sleicher, D., Maron, D. D., Shihab, H. M., Ranasinghe, P. D., Linn, S., Saha, S., Bass, E. B., & Haythornthwaite, J. A. (2014). Meditation programs for psychological stress and wellbeing: a systematic review and meta-analysis. JAMA internal medicine, 174(3), 357–368. https://jamanetwork.com/journals/jamainternalmedicine/fullarticle/1809754

Hoge, E. A., Bui, E., Marques, L., Metcalf, C. A., Morris, L. K., Robinaugh, D. J., Worthington, J. J., Pollack, M. H., & Simon, N. M. (2013). Randomized controlled trial of mindfulness meditation for generalized anxiety disorder: effects on anxiety and stress reactivity. The Journal of clinical psychiatry, 74(8), 786–792.

https://www.psychiatrist.com/jcp/anxiety/randomized-controlled-trial-mindfulness-meditation/

Kasala, E. R., Bodduluru, L. N., Maneti, Y., & Thipparaboina, R. (2014). Effect of meditation on neurophysiological changes in stress mediated depression. Complementary therapies in clinical practice, 20(1), 74–80.

https://www.sciencedirect.com/science/article/abs/pii/S1744388113000674?via%3Dihub

Khanna, A. (n.d.). Why is it important to know your DOSHA? Maharishi Ayurveda website: Https://maharishiayurvedaindia.com/blogs/ayurveda-knowledge-center/why-is-it-important-to-know-your-dosha

Link, R. (2017). 13 Benefits of Yoga That Are Supported by Science. Healthline website:

https://www.healthline.com/nutrition/13-benefits-of-yoga

Link, R. (2019, July 31). What Is the Ayurvedic Diet? Benefits, Downsides, and More. Healthline website: https://www.healthline.com/nutrition/ayurvedic-diet#the-diet

Meditation in Ayurveda - AskDabur. (n.d.). www.dabur.com website:

https://www.dabur.com/daburarogya/ayurveda/arogya-jeevan/meditation-in-ayurveda.aspx

Orme-Johnson, D. W., & Barnes, V. A. (2014). Effects of the transcendental meditation technique on trait anxiety: a meta-analysis of randomized controlled trials. Journal of alternative and complementary medicine (New York, N.Y.), 20(5), 330–341. https://www.liebertpub.com/doi/10.1089/acm.2013.0204

Radloff, M. (n.d.). Sanskrit: The Language of Ayurveda. National Ayurvedic Medical Association website:
https://www.ayurvedanama.org/articles/2019/9/19/sanskrit-the-language-of-ayurveda

Rioux, J., Thomson, C., & Howerter, A. (2014). A Pilot Feasibility Study of Whole-systems Ayurvedic Medicine and Yoga Therapy for Weight Loss. Global advances in health and medicine, 3(1), 28–35.
https://journals.sagepub.com/doi/10.7453/gahmj.2013.084

Roy, A. (2019, May 20). 10 Proven Medical Benefits of Ayurveda. Medlife Blog: Health and Wellness Tips website: https://www.medlife.com/blog/10-proven-medical-benefits-of-ayurveda/

Sharma, S., Puri, S., Agarwal, T., & Sharma, V. (2009). Diets based on Ayurvedic constitution--potential for weight management. Alternative therapies in health and medicine, 15(1), 44–47.

Srour, B., Fezeu, L. K., Kesse-Guyot, E., Allès, B., Méjean, C., Andrianasolo, R. M., Chazelas, E., Deschasaux, M., Hercberg, S., Galan, P., Monteiro, C. A., Julia, C., & Touvier, M. (2019). Ultra-processed food intake and risk of cardiovascular disease: prospective cohort study (NutriNet-Santé). BMJ (Clinical research ed.), 365, l1451. https://www.bmj.com/content/365/bmj.l1451

Thorpe, M. (2020, October 26). 12 Benefits of Meditation. Healthline website: https://www.healthline.com/nutrition/12-benefits-of-meditation#1.-Reduces-stress

Yoga: Methods, types, philosophy, and risks. (n.d.).
https://www.medicalnewstoday.com/ website:

https://www.medicalnewstoday.com/articles/286745

Watts, M. (n.d.). 10 Ways Ayurveda Benefits your Daily Life. Gaiam website:

https://www.gaiam.com/blogs/discover/10-ways-ayurveda-benefits-your-daily-life

What is the relationship between yoga and ayurveda. (n.d.).
https://www.indianyogaassociation.com/ website:
https://www.indianyogaassociation.com/blog/what-is-the-relationship-between-yoga-and-ayurveda.html

9 781638 180380